Introduction 5

Epidemiology and genetics 7

Pathology 15

The clinical picture 25

Treatment of relapses and symptoms 58

Disease-modifying treatment 75

Emerging therapies 98

Special MS populations 106

Lifestyle considerations and the multidisciplinary team 117

Advanced multiple sclerosis 125

Useful resources 131

Index 134

Introduction

Multiple sclerosis (MS) affects people in the most productive period of their lives, affecting quality of life, family and career. MS produces both physical and neuropsychiatric effects, and cognitive decline is an increasingly recognized complication. A lifelong disease, MS also carries with it considerable individual and societal economic burden.

Since the last edition of this book, the diagnostic criteria for MS have been revised and there has been substantial progress in the search for factors that contribute to the development of the disease. These advances, coupled with recent developments in imaging, are helping clinicians to diagnose and potentially treat MS in the earliest phases of the disease. New treatments are now available and many more are in development. With this edition, we hope to emphasize the sense of optimism embodied by current advances in research and treatment.

Historically, the earliest personal account of MS was recorded in the diaries of Frederick D'Este, grandson of King George III. Although his condition was not diagnosed in his lifetime, from 1822 to 1846 he kept a detailed log of his symptoms, which included transient loss of vision, clumsiness of the hands, weakness of the legs, incontinence and dizziness. MS became recognized as a clinicopathological entity around 1870, when Charcot noted a link between the symptoms of MS and nerve damage. Over the next 50 years various hypotheses were promulgated, including an infectious cause, and oligoclonal bands were discovered in the cerebrospinal fluid. By 1950, it was clear that MS was a disease of the central nervous system and by 1960 the beneficial effect of steroids in the management of acute relapses had been identified. By the 1990s the first injectable disease-modifying drugs were in use, and in 2001 criteria for the diagnosis of MS were revolutionized by the incorporation of magnetic resonance imaging (MRI) to demonstrate dissemination of lesions in space and time.

The focus of research is now on finding treatments that will affect the progression of, and potentially reverse, disability. The search for biomarkers that will highlight vulnerable populations is also well under way. While modern therapies are highly effective in preventing

5

relapses and new treatments are evolving rapidly, the holy grail of finding the cause of the disease and the capacity to prevent its development are not yet within our grasp.

In this completely revised edition of *Fast Facts: Multiple Sclerosis* we present the latest evidence on disease pathomechanisms, clinical aspects and modern diagnostic criteria, and review novel therapies that have been recently incorporated into an expanding MS treatment armamentarium. We also emphasize the importance of multidisciplinary management in patients with MS, and with this in mind have written this handbook for the benefit of all healthcare professionals involved in the care of patients with this complex disease.

Multiple sclerosis (MS) is a neurological condition resulting from inflammation within the central nervous system (CNS). This inflammation can affect different sites at different times, producing a variety of symptoms and signs. In the early stages there are periods of relapse and remission, and in most patients a slowly progressive course ensues within one to two decades of disease onset. The cause of MS is unknown, but dysregulation of the immune system is central to the pathogenesis of the disease.

Epidemiology

MS is the leading cause of neurological disability in the young and middle-aged populations of the developed world. 2013 survey figures suggest that it affects around 100 000 people in the UK, 21 000 in Australia and 400 000 in the USA, and an estimated 2.3 million people worldwide. This is likely to be a significant underestimate as there is little published information on populations in many countries.

Prevalence. The number of people with MS in a given population at any one time is usually expressed as cases per 100 000 population. MS is most prevalent in northern European Caucasian populations, especially individuals of Nordic descent, and is notably more prevalent in temperate than equatorial regions. The worldwide prevalence of MS appears to be increasing: this is related to many factors, including increasing diagnostic accuracy, an aging population and a true increase in disease incidence, especially in females. Prevalence rates vary worldwide and in some countries exceed 250 per 100 000. Globally, the median estimated prevalence of MS is 33 per 100 000. Regionally, the median estimated prevalence of MS is greatest in North America and Europe (140 and 108 per 100 000, respectively). The estimated prevalence is 164 per 100 000 people in the UK, 95.6 per 100 000 in Australia and 135 per 100 000 in the USA. Prevalence rates vary significantly both within regions and within countries. Prevalence peaks at age 50.

Incidence. The number of new cases per 100 000 population per year can indicate changes in the risk of a disease within a population, and can signify whether the disease frequency is increasing in a population. It is not affected by changes in survival. The incidence of MS, which peaks at age 30, appears to be rising in both the northern and southern hemispheres, particularly in women. The median estimated global incidence of MS is 2.5 per 100 000 per year, but in some countries incidence rates may exceed 10 per 100 000 per year.

Geo-epidemiology of MS. The prevalence of MS is significantly associated with latitude, particularly in populations of European descent (Figure 1.1). The 'latitudinal gradient' in MS has been confirmed by independent studies in Australia, New Zealand and the USA, with exceptions in Sardinia and northern Scandinavia. In Australia, the prevalence in Tasmania is six times greater than that in

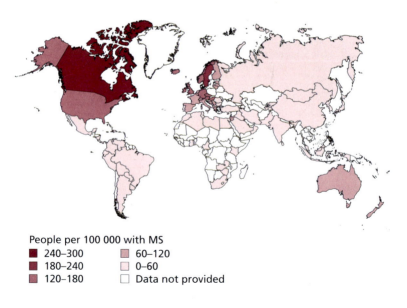

People per 100 000 with MS
- ■ 240–300
- ■ 180–240
- ■ 120–180
- ■ 60–120
- ■ 0–60
- □ Data not provided

Figure 1.1 Geographic distribution of MS, showing a greater prevalence at high latitudes. Source: *Atlas of MS Database*. Multiple Sclerosis International Federation, 2013. www.atlasofms.org

northern Queensland. Genetic variation between geographically discrete populations has been invoked as one explanation for this observation, particularly within the human leukocyte antigen (HLA). However, a statistically significant relationship between MS prevalence and latitude persists in some European populations even after adjustment for HLA-DRB1 allele frequency, supporting a role for environmental factors that vary with latitude (e.g. ultraviolet [UV] light exposure and vitamin D levels).

Sex. MS is more common in women than men, at a ratio of 2–3:1. In Denmark, where an MS registry has been ongoing since 1948, there appears to be an increase in the incidence of MS in women, with a stable rate in the male population. An increasing incidence in females only has also been observed in southern hemisphere populations such as Australia over a similar period.

Environmental risk factors include:
- UV radiation and season of birth
- levels of dietary vitamin D
- Epstein-Barr virus (EBV) infection
- smoking
- migration.

Ultraviolet radiation and season of birth. The latitudinal prevalence gradient for MS may be explained in part by a relationship to exposure to UV radiation from sunlight, as there is an association between low levels of UVB exposure and development of MS. This may explain the 'season of birth effect' whereby those born in spring (April) in countries in the Northern hemisphere have a significantly higher relative risk of developing MS than those born in winter months (October). This may be related to maternal exposure to UV light.

Dietary vitamin D. There is an association between low levels of vitamin D and a number of diseases including MS. UV radiation is the main source of vitamin D; however, populations exposed to limited sunlight but who consume diets rich in fatty fish, a good source of vitamin D, have lower MS prevalence rates than expected for their

9

latitude. While prospective studies have shown that MS risk is lower in groups who take vitamin D supplements regularly, and higher vitamin D levels are associated with lower risk of relapse, the results of large randomized controlled studies in patients with clinically isolated demyelinating syndromes are keenly awaited.

Epstein Barr virus is a double-stranded DNA virus that is transmitted via saliva. EBV does not always cause illness, and early childhood infection with the virus is usually asymptomatic. The acute illness caused by EBV, infectious mononucleosis, often accompanies primary infection in adolescence or young adulthood. Individuals with MS are rarely seronegative for EBV, and there is a strong association between a previous history of infectious mononucleosis and MS, with a twofold greater risk of MS in this group. There also appears to be a relationship between the titers of EBV immunoglobulin G (IgG) and the risk of MS. The nature of the association between EBV and MS is yet to be established, but the infection may trigger or potentiate autoimmunity.

Smoking. The risk of MS is much higher in 'ever smokers' than 'never smokers' and there is a direct link between duration and intensity of smoking. The risk appears to be greater in male (threefold) than female (twofold) smokers. Cultural trends that have led to an increase in the number of female smokers may be contributing to the rising incidence of MS in females.

Migration studies support a relationship between the country of origin and risk of MS. An individual's age at the time of migration from a high prevalence area to one of low prevalence appears to affect the risk for MS, with a critical time period that may extend into early adulthood. Although this observation lends indirect support to the hypothesis that environmental factors contribute to MS risk, the correlation between migration and MS risk is not necessarily maintained when people from communities that do not classically have a high MS prevalence, such as the Japanese, move to areas of high prevalence.

Genetics

No single causative gene for MS has been identified. However, there is
greater risk of developing MS for people with a family member with

this diagnosis (Table 1.1). Concordance between female monozygotic (identical) twins approaches 40%, while dizygotic (non-identical) twins have a concordance rate of approximately 4% and non-twin siblings have a relative risk 15–20 times that of the local population. Although these figures also implicate environmental factors in the genesis of MS, studies of 'non-biological siblings', that is, siblings who share the same environment but have different biological parents, do not suggest an increased risk related solely to environment. It is therefore likely that an individual's genetic background modulates susceptibility to environmental risk factors.

There is a strong association between susceptibility to MS and specific HLA alleles that code for major histocompatibility complex (MHC) class II antigens. These antigens are expressed on antigen-presenting cells (including dendritic cells, macrophages and B lymphocytes). In Caucasians, *HLA-DRB1*1501* has been consistently

TABLE 1.1

Population-based prevalence in relatives of a person with MS

	Prevalence
General population	1/1000
Adoptive siblings	1/1000
First cousin	7/1000
Paternal half sibling	13/1000
Half sibling reared apart	21/1000
Maternal half sibling	24/1000
Full sibling	35/1000
HLA-identical sibling	80/1000
Sibling in consanguineous mating*	90/1000
Child or sibling	197/1000
Offspring of conjugal pair	200/1000
Monozygotic twin	270/1000

*Sibling with same parents, where the parents are related.

associated with MS. It may be that an effect of one gene is modified by several other genes (epistasis). Carrying one copy of this allele (heterozygosity) increases the risk of MS three times, and carrying two copies (homozygosity) increases the risk to six times greater than that of non-carriers. Furthermore, epigenetic modulation of MHC by environmental factors such as vitamin D, smoking, Epstein Barr virus infection and early-life hygiene may modify the effect of allelic variation at this site.

In recent years, a number of other susceptibility loci have been identified, most recently by the International Multiple Sclerosis Genetics Consortium in a study of over 14 000 people with MS that expanded the number of genetic variations associated with MS to

Key points – epidemiology and genetics

- At least 2.3 million people worldwide have been diagnosed with multiple sclerosis (MS).
- MS is more common in women than men (2–3:1), and the incidence of MS in females is rising.
- The prevalence of MS is increasing worldwide, with a greater prevalence in populations of northern European descent.
- There is a 'latitudinal gradient' of MS. In areas of higher latitude (remote from the equator) there is increased prevalence and incidence of people with MS.
- There is an association between low levels of vitamin D and prevalence of MS.
- Most people with MS have been exposed to Epstein–Barr virus (EBV). People who have had infectious mononucleosis have a twofold higher risk of developing MS.
- The rate of MS is higher in smokers than in those who have never smoked.
- MS has a heritable component, but the condition is not related to a single gene (multiple gene interactions are likely to be involved); the human leukocyte antigen (HLA) allele DRB1*1501 has a strong association with MS in Caucasians.

more than 100. Most of the risk alleles associated with MS are related to function of the immune system. An individual's genetic background may also explain the varied response to immunotherapy, and pharmacogenomic studies are ongoing.

Ethnicity. MS is more common in people with northern European ancestry. The incidence is lower in people of Asian/African or South American heritage. People living in the same environment with different ethnicities have different prevalence rates for MS. This highlights the genetic contribution to MS susceptibility.

Key references

Ascherio A, Munger KL, Lünemann JD. The initiation and prevention of multiple sclerosis. *Nat Rev Neurology* 2012;8:602–12.

Dobson R, Giovannoni G, Ramagopalan S. The month of birth effect in multiple sclerosis: systematic review, meta-analysis and effect of latitude. *J Neurol Neurosurg Psychiatry* 2013;84:427–32.

Dyment DA, Ebers GC, Sadovnick AD. Genetics of multiple sclerosis. *Lancet Neurol* 2004;3:104–10.

Ebers GC. Environmental factors and multiple sclerosis. *Lancet Neurol* 2008;7:268–77.

Hurwitz BJ. Analysis of current multiple sclerosis registries. *Neurology* 2011;76(Suppl 1): S7–S13.

International Multiple Sclerosis Genetics Consortium (IMSGC). Analysis of immune-related loci identifies 48 new susceptibility variants for multiple sclerosis. *Nat Genet* 2013;45:1353–60.

Koch-Henriksen N, Soelberg Sørensen P. The changing demographic pattern of multiple sclerosis epidemiology. *Lancet Neurol* 2010;9:520–32.

MSIF. Atlas of MS 2013: Mapping Multiple Sclerosis Around The World. Multiple Sclerosis International Federation, 2013. www.atlasofms.org; www.msif.org/includes/documents/cm_docs/2013/m/msif-atlas-of-ms-2013-report.pdf?f=1; last accessed 12 March 2014.

Pugliatti M, Sotgiu S, Rosati G. The worldwide prevalence of multiple sclerosis. *Clin Neurol Neurosurg* 2002;104:182–91.

Ramagopalan SV, Dobson R, Meier UC, Giovannoni G. Multiple sclerosis: risk factors, prodromes, and potential causal pathways. *Lancet Neurol* 2010;9:727–39.

Scalfari A, Neuhaus A, Degenhardt A et al. The natural history of multiple sclerosis, a geographically based study 10: relapses and long-term disability. *Brain* 2010;133:1914–29.

Simpson S Jr, Blizzard L, Otahal P et al. Latitude is significantly associated with the prevalence of multiple sclerosis: a meta-analysis. *J Neurol Neurosurg Psychiatry* 2011;82:1132–41.

Simpson S Jr, Taylor B, Blizzard L et al. Higher 25-hydroxyvitamin D is associated with lower relapse risk in multiple sclerosis. *Ann Neurol* 2010;68:193–203.

Tremlett H, Zhao Y, Rieckmann P, Hutchinson M. New perspectives in the natural history of multiple sclerosis. *Neurology* 2010;74:2005.

Willer CJ, Dyment DA, Sadovnick AD et al. Timing of birth and risk of multiple sclerosis: population-based study. *BMJ* 2005;330:120.

The neuropathological examination of affected brain and spinal cord tissue has driven multiple sclerosis (MS) research for more than 170 years, and in large part has shaped concepts of pathogenesis, tissue injury and repair. In contrast to gray matter, which contains neural cell bodies, white matter predominantly contains myelinated axon tracts. MS is characterized by the presence of multifocal lesions or 'plaques', predominantly in the white matter, which exhibit myelin destruction, perivascular inflammation and relative preservation of axons.

The condition is traditionally regarded as a T-cell-mediated inflammatory demyelinating disease, initiated outside the central nervous system (CNS) by loss of tolerance to one, or a number of, CNS antigen(s). This hypothesis is now regarded as an oversimplification, and neuropathological, biomarker and treatment studies have implicated B cells, regulatory T cells and factors within the CNS as critical pathophysiological determinants.

Lesion distribution

The number, size and distribution of lesions vary widely amongst individuals with MS. In early disease most patients have small circumscribed lesions that typically occur in the periventricular and subcortical white matter, corpus callosum, optic nerves, cerebellum and spinal cord (Figure 2.1). Predominant involvement of the spinal cord and optic nerves with minimal hemispheric pathology is also observed in a proportion of patients, who may represent a distinct MS subset.

Although disease may be macroscopically confined to the white matter, careful neuropathological evaluation reveals focal cortical and deep gray matter lesions in almost all patients with MS (Figure 2.2). Rarely, patients present with massive ('tumefactive') hemispheric lesions that are mistaken for primary brain neoplasms until typical pathological changes of MS are identified on biopsy tissue.

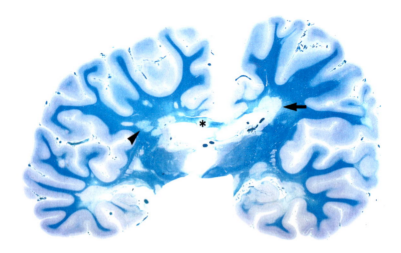

Figure 2.1 Whole brain coronal section from a patient with secondary progressive MS. Typical small chronic lesions are present in the corpus callosum (asterisk) and periventricular white matter (arrow) of both hemispheres. Remyelinated lesions, which stain palely for myelin, are also present (arrowhead). Small leukocortical lesions are visible at higher power in both hemispheres. Luxol fast-blue.

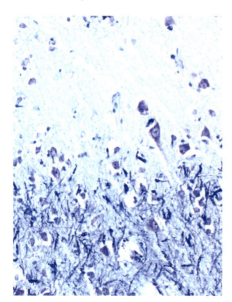

Figure 2.2 The edge of a chronically demyelinated cortical lesion, which also involves the adjacent white matter, in a patient with secondary progressive MS. Note the reduction in neuronal density in the demyelinated (upper) zone of gray matter. Luxol fast-blue cresyl violet.

Many MS lesions are associated with cerebral vessels, and some contain a small central vein. However, these are often 'satellite' extensions of a larger lesion without any apparent vascular relationship; the innumerable perivenular inflammatory lesions that characterize acute disseminated encephalomyelitis (ADEM) and the animal model experimental allergic encephalomyelitis (EAE) are largely absent in MS.

Chronic lesions

Well-circumscribed, chronic, hypocellular, white matter plaques predominate in most patients with longstanding MS. The majority of these lesions are devoid of myelin and exhibit *relative* axonal preservation (Figure 2.3). Few mature oligodendrocytes are present, and there is variable astrocytic proliferation and gliosis. A proportion of chronic lesions may have a fringe of thin myelin sheaths at the plaque border, representing remyelination. Conversely, active breakdown of myelin sheaths may be present in the edge of slowly

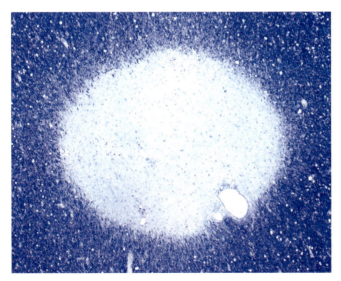

Figure 2.3 A small, well-circumscribed lesion in the deep white matter in a patient with established MS. The lesion is completely devoid of myelin, has relatively well-preserved axons and exhibits a moderate degree of astrogliosis. Luxol fast-blue.

expanding chronic plaques (chronic active plaques), a frequent finding in some patients with secondary progressive MS.

Acute lesions: implications for pathogenesis

The hallmark of the acute MS lesion is the abrupt appearance of large numbers of activated microglia and macrophages, outnumbering lymphocytes by at least 10–20 times, in concert with the start of myelin breakdown and focal disruption of the blood–brain barrier. Active lesions, which predominate in early relapsing MS, are defined pathologically by the presence of partially myelinated axons in tissue infiltrated by macrophages. When stained with Luxol fast-blue (a stain for myelin), these macrophages are found to contain myelin particles that are immunoreactive for myelin proteins (Figure 2.4). Most such macrophages, which display enhanced expression of CD45 and major histocompatibility complex (MHC) class II antigens, appear in sheets and are thought to derive primarily from resident microglia, rather than circulating monocytes.

The nature of the macrophage 'attack' on apparently normal myelin is unclear. In the most widely accepted paradigm, phagocytic activity is directed by myelin-specific T cells in perivascular cuffs and, in lesser

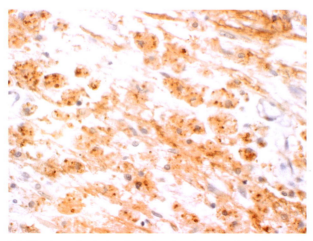

Figure 2.4 Classic active lesion in early relapsing MS. Partially myelinated axons are infiltrated by numerous macrophages containing particles that immunostain positively for myelin. Myelin-oligodendrocyte glycoprotein.

numbers, diffusely infiltrating the parenchyma within such lesions. The process is facilitated by the secretion of injurious toxins including tumor necrosis factor (TNF)-α, reactive oxygen species and proteolytic enzymes. This hypothesis has been challenged by the neuropathological interrogation of ultra-acute (newly forming) MS lesions, which are characterized by extensive loss of oligodendrocytes without significant T-cell infiltrates. Whatever the cause, myelin loss from axons proceeds rapidly and is usually complete within 2 weeks from symptom onset. Lesions examined during this time show a variable reduction in oligodendrocyte numbers and evidence of at least modest axonal injury.

Normal conduction in surviving axons is disrupted by the inflammatory milieu and demyelination, resulting in slowed impulse conduction. A proportion of demyelinated fibers are unable to support impulse conduction, in part because of a low density of sodium channels in the axon membrane, resulting in 'conduction block' and the development of neurological symptoms. Compensatory alterations in the redistribution of ion channels (sodium/potassium) underlie responses to drugs such as potassium channel blockers (e.g. fampridine). Paradoxically, it is precisely these physiological changes that may contribute to increased metabolic 'stress', which in turn may hasten axonal damage.

The periplaque white matter

The periplaque white matter is the zone immediately surrounding acute and chronic MS lesions, and is characterized by the presence of activated microglia (which may form specific elongated 'nodules' or aggregates; Figure 2.5), perivascular T-cell cuffs and proliferating oligodendrocytes. While poorly defined, the molecular events that take place in the periplaque white matter are probably critical to both lesion formation and repair.

Remyelination

Recovery from relapses is in part mediated by remyelination, the process by which denuded axons are enveloped by new myelin sheaths (Figures 2.6 and 2.7). New myelin is laid down by a population of

19

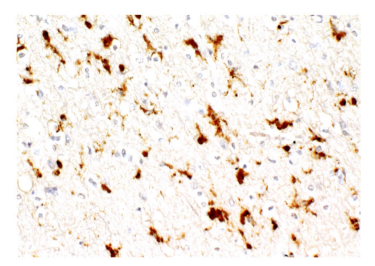

Figure 2.5 Extensive microglial activation in the normally myelinated periplaque white matter of a patient with secondary progressive MS. Occasionally, microglia in the periplaque white matter may form elongated nodules, possibly around short axon segments that are immunoreactive for complement (C3d). CD68.

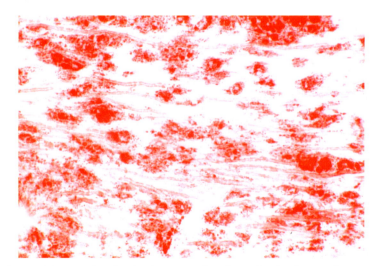

Figure 2.6 Remyelination begins soon after demyelination is complete in the early relapsing phase of MS. Thinly (re)myelinated axons are interspersed by numerous lipid-laden macrophages in this recently active spinal cord lesion. Oil Red O.

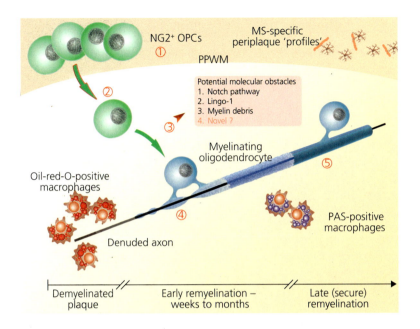

Figure 2.7 Principal pathological features of early/late remyelination. In early relapsing MS, the process of remyelination begins soon after a demyelinating event, indicated here by the presence of Oil-red-O-positive macrophages. The circled numbers represent potential sites for dysregulation of remyelination: NG2+ oligodendrocyte progenitor cells (OPCs) (1) proliferate in periplaque white matter (PPWM) surrounding recently demyelinated tissue and (2) migrate into the plaque. Here, they (3) differentiate into myelinating oligodendrocytes that (4) ensheath denuded axons with new myelin lamellae. Neuropathological examination at this time may reveal older PAS-positive macrophages. With time, fusion of myelin lamellae promotes (5) the formation of compact myelin.

oligodendrocytes that appears within lesions only days after an episode of acute inflammatory demyelination. These myelinating cells are derived from oligodendrocyte progenitor cells, which must migrate from the periplaque white matter and mature before commencing the process of axon ensheathment.

Although remyelination is the default response to demyelination in early relapsing disease, the process progressively fails with advancing

21

disease and age in many patients. The subsequent loss of myelin-associated trophic signals contributes to axonal degeneration and the accrual of irreversible disability. The molecular mechanisms that underpin remyelination failure are yet to be fully elucidated, and current MS therapies, which effectively target inflammatory pathology in early disease, do not promote endogenous repair mechanisms or arrest disease progression. A Phase II randomized controlled trial of anti-LINGO1, a humanized monoclonal antibody designed to promote remyelination and restore function, is currently under way.

'Neurodegeneration' and gray matter lesions

Although myelin appears to be 'targeted' in MS lesions, focal and diffuse axonal loss is present in the white matter of patients with relapsing and progressive forms of the disease. Diffuse white matter axonal loss becomes most prominent in longstanding disease, and is accompanied by diffuse activation of microglia and the presence of scattered perivascular T-cell cuffs. This so-called neurodegenerative component of MS correlates strongly with the development of irreversible disability and MRI measures such as whole-brain atrophy.

While MS is traditionally regarded as a white matter disease, prominent demyelination, neuro-axonal injury and loss of synapses are present in the cortex and deep gray matter of patients with longstanding disease and underpin the cognitive and, to a lesser extent, motor dysfunction that characterizes this phase of the condition.

Focal gray matter lesions are less inflammatory than their white matter counterparts, likely a reflection of reduced myelin density in the gray matter rather than any fundamental difference in lesion pathogenesis. Focal cortical lesions are, however, often topographically related to meningeal lymphoid aggregates, implicating a local effect of T or B cells. A recent analysis of brain biopsies from patients with clinically isolated events (see Chapter 3) suggests that focal cortical pathology may also be common in early disease. Concordant with this finding, neuroimaging studies indicate that brain volume loss preferentially occurs in the gray matter in early relapsing MS.

Key points – pathology

- Early relapsing MS is a multifocal inflammatory demyelinating disease that affects both the white and gray matter.
- Although still considered to be an organ-specific autoimmune disease, loss of myelin-forming oligodendrocytes in newly forming MS lesions is a critical event that may trigger or amplify the inflammatory cascade that characterizes active demyelination.
- Resolution of inflammation, restoration of axonal impulse propagation and remyelination mediate recovery from discrete clinical relapses in early disease.
- Molecular reorganization of demyelinated axon membranes, characterized by a greater than normal sodium channel density, permits the restoration of continuous impulse propagation in non-remyelinated fibers.
- As the disease advances, the pathological complexity of MS increases. Multifocal adaptive inflammation is progressively replaced by a diffuse 'degenerative' phase, although these two facets of MS neuropathology are probably inextricably linked.
- Current therapies effectively target the inflammatory pathology that peaks in early disease, but fail to arrest the progression of established 'neurodegeneration' or promote endogenous repair mechanisms such as remyelination.

Key references

Barnett MH, Prineas JW. Relapsing and remitting multiple sclerosis: pathology of the newly forming lesion. *Ann Neurol* 2004;55:458–68.

Fancy SP, Kotter MR, Harrington EP et al. Overcoming remyelination failure in multiple sclerosis and other myelin disorders. *Exp Neurol* 2010;225:18–23.

Hohlfeld R, Wekerle H. Autoimmune concepts of multiple sclerosis as a basis for selective immunotherapy: from pipe dreams to (therapeutic) pipelines. *Proc Natl Acad Sci USA* 2004;101(Suppl2):14599–606.

Lucchinetti CF, Popescu BF, Bunyan RF et al. Inflammatory cortical demyelination in early multiple sclerosis. *N Engl J Med* 2011;365:2188–97.

Prineas JW, Kwon EE, Cho ES et al. Immunopathology of secondary-progressive multiple sclerosis. *Ann Neurol* 2001;50:646–57.

Redford EJ, Kapoor R, Smith KJ. Nitric oxide donors reversibly block axonal conduction: demyelinated axons are especially susceptible. *Brain* 1997;120(Pt 12):2149–57.

Multiple sclerosis (MS) is an inflammatory demyelinating disease that affects multiple sites across the central nervous system (CNS). The clinical phenotype of MS depends largely on the location of inflammatory lesions, resulting in a broad spectrum of symptoms and signs. While the majority of individual lesions, particularly within the cerebral hemispheres, are asymptomatic, pathology in 'eloquent' areas such as the optic nerve, spinal cord and brainstem is usually accompanied by a relevant clinical syndrome.

Definitions

Clinically isolated syndrome. The first presentation of demyelination is termed a clinically isolated syndrome (CIS). People with these presentations do not have *clinically definite* MS; however, the presence of asymptomatic demyelinating lesions on MRI at the time of a CIS predicts a high likelihood of developing clinically definite MS (approximately 90% over 1–2 decades).

Clinically definite MS. A person has clinically definite MS when there is objective clinical evidence of lesion dissemination in time (DIT) and space (DIS). The second clinical episode must occur in a different site from the original lesion at least 1 month later. When reviewing a patient with CIS or MS, a detailed neurological history and examination must be taken to search for evidence of new symptoms or signs of CNS demyelination. Importantly, the incorporation of MRI into modern diagnostic criteria permits a diagnosis of MS to be made in some patients at the time of a CIS.

Types of multiple sclerosis

It is important to define the subtype of MS, as this will guide prognosis and choice of disease-modifying therapy. For example, therapies that reduce the frequency and severity of relapses may not be helpful to people with progressive disease. As all of the available treatments have potential side effects, all patients should be provided with a risk–benefit analysis appropriate to their MS subtype. The recognized patterns of MS are:

- relapsing remitting
- secondary progressive
- primary progressive
- progressive relapsing
- benign.

Relapsing remitting disease is the most common form of MS, accounting for 65–70% of patients. Relapsing remitting MS is characterized by periods of acute neurological disturbance (relapses), which last for at least 24 hours and are not attributable to other causes such as infection or changes in core temperature. These relapses must occur after more than 30 days of clinical stability, and the neurological deficit must be established objectively by clinical evaluation (history and/or examination).

In early disease, recovery after a relapse (remission) is often near complete, but incomplete recovery is common in established disease and in these instances patients with MS often accrue disability with each successive relapse (Figure 3.1).

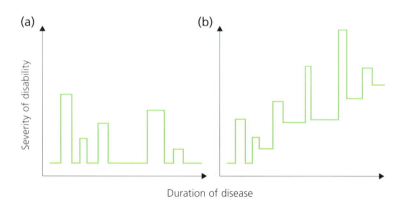

Figure 3.1 The two patterns of relapsing remitting disease: (a) relapses with return to normal neurological function; (b) relapsing disease with stepwise, accumulated disability.

Secondary progressive disease. In most cases (up to 75% of people with relapsing remitting disease) there is an eventual progression to the secondary progressive phase of MS. This is defined as an initial relapsing remitting disease course followed by progression with or without occasional relapses, minor remissions and plateaus (Figure 3.2). Risk factors for progression to secondary progressive MS are shown in Table 3.1. The progression of disease from relapsing remitting to the secondary progressive stage is usually noted retrospectively, for example when a patient with MS has accumulated disability over 6–12 months without any discrete episodes of relapse. Neuroaxonal loss without any 'overt' features of inflammation (clinical or radiological) is thought to underlie this phase of MS (Figure 3.3).

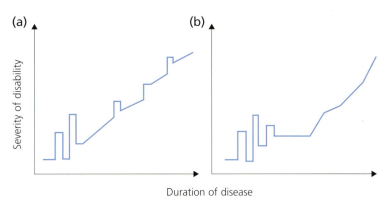

Figure 3.2 In secondary progressive MS, patients (a) may or (b) may not continue to have relapses.

TABLE 3.1

Risk factors associated with progression to secondary progressive MS

- Older age at disease onset
- Short interval between the first and second relapses
- Higher and increasing T2 lesion load
- Motor deficit with incomplete recovery

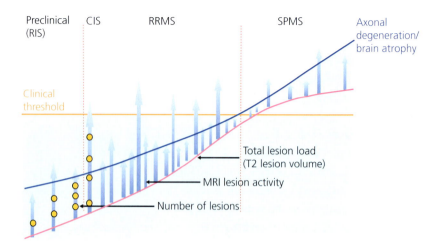

Figure 3.3 The natural history of MS. Silent inflammatory activity almost certainly begins before the first clinical event (CIS). Lesions compatible with inflammatory demyelination discovered incidentally by MRI during the preclinical phase are termed the radiologically isolated syndrome (RIS). The incorporation of MRI into modern diagnostic criteria permits determination of dissemination in time (DIT), in the absence of a second clinical event, when new T2 (or contrast-enhancing) lesions are present on follow-up imaging. The 2010 McDonald criteria permit a diagnosis of MS to be made at the time of a CIS if there are both enhancing and non-enhancing lesions (indicating DIT) on MRI. In parallel with the development of relapses and new T2 lesions, there is progressive loss of axons, neurons and synapses from the earliest phases of the disease, which manifests clinically with secondary progression when neuroaxonal reserves are exhausted, indicated here by the 'clinical threshold'. In this secondary progressive phase of MS, acute discrete inflammatory events (contrast-enhancing lesions, new T2 lesions) wane and progressive brain atrophy dominates the MRI picture. RRMS, relapsing remitting MS; SPMS, secondary progressive MS.

Primary progressive disease comprises approximately 10–15% of patients with MS. It does not present with discrete relapses, but a gradual progression of disability, often attributable to spinal motor involvement (Figure 3.4). Primary progressive MS typically has a later onset than relapsing remitting MS.

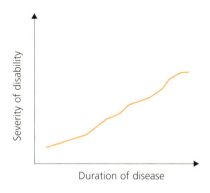

Figure 3.4 Typical pattern of progressive disability in primary progressive disease.

Progressive relapsing disease. Many texts do not recognize this entity, but in the authors' experience a small number of patients present with gradually progressive disease onto which are 'superimposed' periods of worsening that may be steroid responsive (Figure 3.5). While a clear history of discrete relapsing remitting symptoms may be lacking in these patients, a proportion may have acute (gadolinium-enhancing) MRI lesions and respond to immunomodulatory therapies. Progressive relapsing disease should therefore be differentiated from primary and secondary progressive disease. Recently, 'active' (clinical relapses or new/enhancing MRI lesions) and 'inactive' phenotypes of progressive MS have been proposed by an international working group.

Benign MS is a further classification, applicable to approximately 5–8% of patients. It is usually defined by a lack of accrued disability after more than 20 years' disease duration. It is difficult to predict

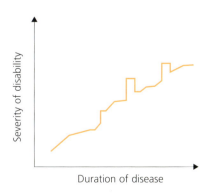

Figure 3.5 Pattern of disease in progressive relapsing multiple sclerosis – progression of disability with 'superimposed' periods of worsening.

which patients will have a benign course at disease onset and it is invariably a retrospective diagnosis.

Patient history

Medical history. People with MS do not always seek medical attention in the early phase of the disease, especially when the sensory pathways are affected in isolation or if symptoms such as visual blurring are mild and temporary. However, it is important at presentation to determine whether a patient presenting with an apparent CIS has experienced a prior remitting neurological disturbance of any sort (Table 3.2).

L'hermitte's sign is an unpleasant paroxysmal sensation, often described as an electric shock radiating along the spine and into the limbs when the neck is flexed. This indicates that there is an 'irritative' lesion at the level of the cervical cord and is thought to be due to stretching of hyperexcitable neurons in the dorsal column. It is common in MS, but can be associated with other causes of cervical spinal cord disease (e.g. cord compression, vitamin B_{12} deficiency, radiation myelopathy).

TABLE 3.2

Useful questions for ascertaining prior neurological disturbances

Have you ever experienced numbness or heaviness in any of your limbs, particularly in association with changes in bladder or bowel function that went away before you sought medical help?

Have you ever experienced numbness or a feeling of a tight band across your trunk?

Have you ever had a painful eye or a loss of vision which lasted for a few days or weeks?

Has your color vision ever been affected?

Have you ever had double vision that lasted for more than a day?

Have you ever had vertigo or balance difficulties (ataxia) that lasted for more than a few days?

Uhthoff's phenomenon is the worsening of neurological symptoms as the patient's core body temperature increases; for example, increased visual blurring after a hot shower or a worsening of pre-existing limb weakness in high ambient temperatures.

Other autoimmune diseases. As there is an association between MS and other autoimmune diseases such as thyroid disease, diabetes mellitus, vitiligo and inflammatory bowel disease, it is important to include questions about these when taking a history.

Family history. The risk of MS rises with increasing genetic proximity to an affected individual (see Table 1.1, page 11). It is therefore important to document any family history of MS or autoimmune diseases (which are often familial). The onset of MS tends to be earlier in people with familial MS.

Social history. Smoking is a risk factor for MS. It is also important to establish country of origin and time of migration when trying to establish the likelihood of MS (see Chapter 1).

Signs and symptoms

MS manifests with symptoms or signs that arise from focal inflammatory lesions within the CNS. These can be localized by taking a thorough history and by clinical examination. The symptoms associated with a MS relapse usually evolve over 24 to 48 hours and persist for at least 24 hours, often improving gradually over subsequent days and weeks. Although 'eloquent' regions of the CNS, such as the spinal cord, optic nerve and brainstem, are more likely to result in symptoms (Table 3.3), the spectrum of presenting symptoms associated with demyelination is broad. These may include any cranial nerve palsy; facial myokymia; trigeminal or glossopharyngeal neuralgia; specific spinal syndromes such as deafferented limb and Browne–Sequard syndrome; and seizures. However, only a minority of new lesions (approximately 1 in 10) in the hemispheric deep white matter is symptomatic.

Relapse risk may be heightened up to threefold by recent urinary or respiratory tract infections, or other viral infections, which should be

TABLE 3.3

MS symptoms at presentation and during the course of the disease

	Presenting (%)	During course (%)
Visual/oculomotor	49	100
Paresis	43	88
Paresthesias	41	87
Incoordination	23	82
Genitourinary–bowel	10	63
Cerebral	4	39

documented. Relapses must be differentiated from physiological 'pseudo-relapses' that may occur in the context of infection-related fever. A history of recent vaccination may also be relevant, although prospective studies have not identified a relationship between common vaccines, such as influenza and hepatitis B, and MS relapse.

Loss of visual acuity or color vision often occurs due to inflammatory demyelination in the anterior optic pathways. Optic neuritis, which is retrobulbar in at least two-thirds of cases, results in a reduction in visual acuity accompanied by pain on eye movement. Findings include a visual field defect that is usually paracentral (although any pattern of field loss may occur) and an abnormal pupillary response to light (relative afferent pupillary defect – RAPD). Rarely, anterior optic neuritis results in visible swelling of the optic disc (papillitis), but gross swelling should raise suspicion of an alternative cause. The majority of patients recover their vision over a median period of about 8 weeks. The optic disc becomes pale after many weeks, reflecting loss of axons and their replacement with glial tissue and loss of small capillaries within the nerve.

Internuclear ophthalmoplegia (INO) is a characteristic but not pathognomonic sign of MS caused by a lesion within the ipsilateral fibers of the medial longitudinal fasciculus in the brainstem. INO is

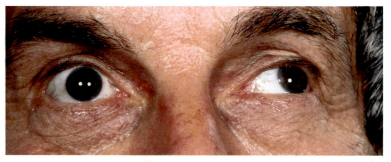

Figure 3.6 Right internuclear ophthalmoplegia. On attempted lateral gaze the patient displays nystagmus in the left (abducting) eye and impaired adduction of the right eye.

often asymptomatic, but patients may complain of diplopia or blurring of vision on lateral gaze. Careful examination of the patient's saccadic eye movements reveals failure of adduction ipsilateral to the lesion and gaze-evoked nystagmus affecting the contralateral abducting eye (Figure 3.6).

Incoordination. Lesions affecting the brainstem and cerebellar pathways are common in patients with MS, and can lead to poor coordination. This can be reflected in an ataxic gait, dysarthria or dysmetria.

Gait problems. People with MS may have a spastic gait, a broad-based ataxic gait or both, depending on the principal site(s) of pathology. Balance is commonly affected. Gait abnormalities can be due to cerebellar, visual, motor or sensory dysfunction.

Speech and swallowing difficulties. Patients may complain of slurred speech. This is most commonly due to involvement of the cerebellum and/or brainstem connections. Swallowing difficulties for solids and/or liquids can occur at any time, although they are typically more common with advanced disease.

Spasticity arises following the loss of inhibitory input from the brain on spinal cord reflexes, resulting in co-contraction of antagonist and agonist muscles. This may manifest as painful spasms, cramps, stiffness and clonus. Both weakness and spasticity contribute to the development of disability.

Other postural/movement problems. Paroxysmal short-lived (less than 60 seconds) disorders of posture/movement (choreo-athetoid/dystonic) may be a sign of ephaptic discharges ('cross talk'), often localized in the brainstem. These need to be distinguished from epileptic discharges, though both may respond to anticonvulsant therapy.

Paresis (motor). Patients may complain of weakness in either the upper or lower limbs, more commonly the latter. The weakness is typically pyramidal in pattern leading to weaker extensor muscles in the upper limbs and weaker flexor muscles in the lower limbs.

Sensory symptoms. Patients may complain of numbness, paresthesias and dysesthesias. Burning discomfort and painful hypersensitivity to touch (allodynia) or temperature frequently occur when demyelination occurs in the spinothalamic pathways.

Pain. Paroxysmal pain, such as trigeminal or glossopharyngeal neuralgia, is not uncommon. Trigeminal neuralgia in MS may be clinically indistinguishable from idiopathic trigeminal neuralgia, but is due to inflammatory demyelination at the fifth cranial nerve root entry zone within the pons rather than irritative pathology of the peripheral (extrapontine) portion of the nerve. Truncal band-like discomfort or pain, often referred to by patients as 'the MS hug', results from spinal cord involvement. Neuropathic pain is also common in patients with MS and can erroneously be mistaken for 'peripheral' compressive neuropathic syndromes such as carpal tunnel syndrome or lumbosacral radiculopathy.

Genitourinary problems. Urinary symptoms include frequency, urgency, urge incontinence, incomplete emptying or retention, and recurrent urinary tract infections. These symptoms should be initially investigated with pre- and post-void bladder ultrasound to assess the urinary residual volume, which will guide the implementation of an appropriate treatment strategy (Figure 3.7).

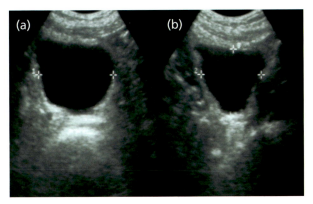

Figure 3.7 Ultrasound scans showing the bladder (a) before voiding and (b) after voiding, with a large residual volume. The cursors (+) mark the bladder-wall boundaries.

Bladder dysfunction includes:
- an inability to store the normal amount of urine
- incomplete emptying
- mismatch of emptying and storing.

Urinary frequency, urgency and urge incontinence reflect detrusor muscle hyperactivity, which is usually due to disruption of voluntary and supraspinal control of voiding by spinal cord pathology above the lumbosacral level. The detrusor stretch reflex is normally activated, signaling the need to urinate, when the bladder contains 300–400 mL of urine. In patients with detrusor hyperactivity, as little as 50–100 mL can activate the detrusor muscle.

Less frequently, the external sphincter fails to relax when the detrusor muscle is contracting, and the patient may experience incomplete emptying despite frequent urination. Retaining urine increases the risk of recurrent urinary tract infection, which may be the main presentation of bladder dysfunction in MS.

Bowel problems. Constipation is a common disturbance in the later stages of the disease. While it commonly reflects spinal disease, constipation can be exacerbated by medications and reduced mobility. Medications that disturb bowel function include antispasmodics, tricyclic antidepressants, anticholinergics and opioids.

Cognitive impairment is a frequent accompaniment of longstanding MS, but can begin in the early relapsing phase of the disease in some patients and is a significant contributor to loss of work and income. Patients with MS are particularly vulnerable to 'subcortical' deficits in information processing and spatial recall. Recent pathological studies have demonstrated a significant burden of cortical and deep gray matter involvement in MS, even at the CIS stage. Volumetric MRI, which demonstrates both cortical and deep gray matter atrophy in MS, and advanced techniques such as magnetization transfer imaging have confirmed a robust correlation of gray matter pathology and cognitive impairment.

It is important to assess and monitor cognition from the time of diagnosis, and practical tools applicable in clinical practice have been developed for this purpose.

Mood disorders. Depression is common and can be an early indicator of cognitive impairment. Patients with MS are up to four times more likely to experience at least one major depressive episode than the general population.

Sexual function can be impaired in people with MS due to both physical and psychological effects of the condition. People with MS may struggle with altered body image, and personal relationships may be affected by the diagnosis and subsequent illness. Individuals may experience altered genital sensation, and disability may affect their ability to engage in intercourse. These issues should be proactively explored by the patient's neurologist or specialist nurse, with discussion of treatment options or practical solutions.

Other symptoms common in MS include fatigue, tremor and pain, which are covered in more detail in the treatment chapter.

Investigations

Table 3.4 provides an overview of the investigations employed in the work up for MS.

TABLE 3.4

Multiple sclerosis investigations

- MRI (± gadolinium) of brain ± spinal cord
- Cerebrospinal fluid
  - cell count
  - protein
  - oligoclonal immunoglobulin G (immunofixation electrophoresis)
- Bloods
  - oligoclonal immunoglobulin G (immunofixation electrophoresis)
  - FBC, ESR, ANA, ANCA, RF, complement, vitamin B_{12}, ACE
  - Antibodies to dsDNA, ENA and phospholipid- and beta-2-GP1.
  - NMO-IgG / AQP-4 antibody
- Visual evoked potentials

ACE, angiotensin-converting enzyme; ANA, antinuclear antibody; ANCA, antineutrophil cytoplasmic antibody; AQP-4, aquaporin 4; ENA; extractable nuclear antigen; ESR, erythrocyte sedimentation rate; FBC, full blood count; GP, glycoprotein; Ig, immunoglobulin; NMO, neuromyelitis optica; RF, rheumatoid factor. Adapted from Wakerley B et al. 2012.

Magnetic resonance imaging remains the most important investigation in the diagnosis and monitoring of MS. White matter lesions are best visualized on T2-weighted and fluid attenuated inversion recovery (FLAIR) sequences. Active inflammation is best seen on enhanced T1-weighted images. Although the abnormalities found on MRI scans – particularly those seen on a single examination – are not specific for the disease, certain combinations of findings on cerebral MRI have a high specificity for MS (Figure 3.8).

Characteristic supratentorial sites include the periventricular region (where lesions are often ovoid or flame-shaped), corpus callosum and juxtacortical areas of the brain. The presence of infratentorial lesions (in the brainstem, cerebellum, cerebellar peduncles and spinal cord) is typical, and helpful in excluding differential diagnoses such as microvascular ischemia.

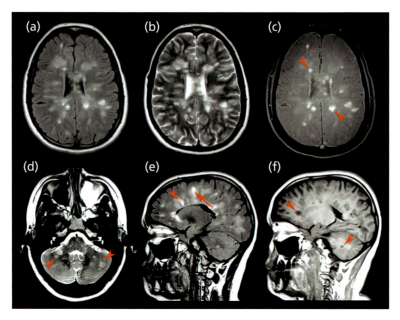

Figure 3.8 MRI scans from an 18-year-old female with highly active relapsing remitting MS and an Expanded Disability Status Score of 2.5. She had experienced increased fatigue and new numbness and clumsiness of her right arm and leg. MS had been diagnosed only 8 months earlier when she presented with left facial numbness. The MRI was acquired using the following pulse sequences: (a) axial fluid-attenuated inversion recovery (FLAIR); (b) axial T2-weighted imaging; (c) axial contrast-enhanced T1-weighted imaging; (d) axial T2-weighted imaging, showing involvement of the posterior fossa structures (arrowheads), which is highly suggestive of MS; (e) sagittal FLAIR, showing typical globular (arrow) and pericallosal (arrowhead) lesions; (f) sagittal T1-weighted imaging. Many, but not all, of the MS lesions are enhanced (examples indicated by arrowheads in [c]), signifying breakdown of the blood–brain barrier and active inflammation. Hypointensities on the T1-weighted images (arrowheads in [f]) could reflect edema and inflammation in acute lesions, or severe axonal injury in chronic lesions. Many lesions have different appearances on images obtained by different sequences, regardless of their enhancement status. This variable pattern is characteristic of MS. Images courtesy of Dr J Frith.

Followed over time, MRI scans in MS typically 'wax and wane', with the emergence of new lesions and the involution of older lesions.

The majority of new lesions exhibit gadolinium enhancement for a
short period (2–6 weeks), reflecting breakdown of the blood–brain
barrier associated with foci of inflammatory demyelination. Acute
lesions are usually iso-intense or hypo-intense (reflecting inflammation
and edema) on unenhanced T1-weighted sequences. Some of these
lesions will remain permanently hypo-intense (T1 'black holes'),
reflecting significant axonal destruction. However, conventional MRI
sequences do not provide specific pathological information about
individual lesions, particularly with regard to the extent of repair/
remyelination. Advanced MRI techniques, including magnetization
transfer imaging (MTI), diffusion tensor imaging (DTI), magnetic
resonance spectroscopy (MRS) and 'myelin water imaging', may
provide specific pathological data in the future.

Spinal cord lesions, which are usually eccentric, dorsal and
span less than two vertebral segments (Figure 3.9), exhibit similar
characteristics on MRI to brain MS lesions. However, spinal lesions
may be subtle, and newer sequences such as short time inversion
recovery (STIR) may be more sensitive than conventional T2-weighted
sequences. MS spinal cord lesions may involve the central gray

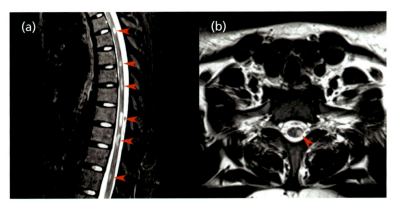

Figure 3.9 Spinal imaging in MS: (a) sagittal short time inversion recovery
(STIR) imaging through the thoracolumbar spine shows at least six short
segment lesions (arrowheads) in a 27-year-old female with relapsing
remitting disease; (b) axial T2-weighted imaging through one of the
thoracic cord lesions shows the typical eccentric location (arrowhead)
within the cord. Images courtesy of Dr Y Barnett.

matter, although less commonly than in conditions such as NMO or ADEM. Chronic spinal cord lesions may be associated with focal atrophy.

Recent studies have demonstrated tight correlation between loss of cortical and deep gray matter volume with cognitive and motor outcomes in MS, highlighting the importance of gray matter pathology. Advances in volumetric MRI, resulting in the accurate segmentation of gray and white matter and estimation of volume changes over time, are now being incorporated into multinational MS clinical trials. The development of new sequences, such as double inversion recovery (DIR) and phase-sensitive inversion recovery (PSIR), allows clinicians and researchers to demonstrate cortical MS lesions, albeit with a sensitivity of only 20–30% (relative to histopathological assessment). Ultra-high-field (7T) MRI may also be a helpful tool in demonstrating cortical pathology, particularly subpial lesions, in the future.

Increasingly, MRI has a role in monitoring for complications of newer immunosuppressive therapies; in particular, progressive multifocal leukoencephalopathy (PML) may rarely complicate treatment with natalizumab, and frequent MRI scans, particularly in patients with serologic evidence of exposure to the causative JC virus (a type of human polyomavirus), may be necessary.

Blood tests (see Table 3.4). It is important to look for other conditions that may mimic MS (see 'Differential diagnosis', page 43). These blood tests are normal/negative in MS, but in patients with MS mimics they may reveal evidence of:
- systemic markers of inflammation (raised C-reactive protein, erythrocyte sedimentation rate, antinuclear antibody, anti-neutrophil cytoplasmic antibody tests)
- other primary demyelinating disease (NMO-IgG / aquaporin 4 antibodies)
- other causes of CNS inflammation (ENA, dsDNA antibodies, antiphospholipid and beta-2-GP1 antibodies).

Significant elevation of serum angiotensin-converting enzyme (ACE) is a relatively specific but insensitive marker of sarcoidosis and should be checked in clinically appropriate cases.

Cerebrospinal fluid. The CSF in patients with MS commonly has a normal or moderately elevated protein content and exhibits a mild inflammatory reaction (typically lymphocytes < 50 cells/dL).

CSF oligoclonal bands. When CSF or serum is passed along an electrical current (electrophoresis), the proteins separate out according to their weight and charge. If there are immunoglobulins (Ig) in this fluid, they will separate out into oligoclonal bands that have a recognizable pattern. The presence of oligoclonal bands in the CSF, *but not the serum*, is consistent with intrathecal IgG synthesis and is found in more than 95% of patients with MS (Figure 3.10). However, CSF-specific oligoclonal bands may be present in other immune-mediated neurological conditions (such as the paraneoplastic or auto-antibody-mediated encephalitides) and in some CNS infections (such as neuroborreliosis). They are usually absent in ADEM, NMO and systemic disease with CNS manifestations. CSF examination should be reserved for patients with atypical clinical presentations or unusual MRI features.

Electrophysiology. Characteristic abnormalities of visual, somatosensory or brainstem evoked potentials may be helpful in confirming that the lesions are disseminated in space in cases where the clinical findings and MRI are not diagnostic. Delayed conduction

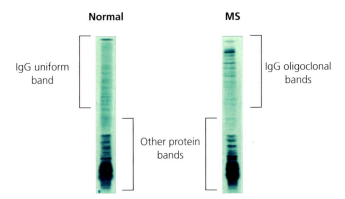

Figure 3.10 Cerebrospinal fluid electrophoresis reveals distinctive oligoclonal immunoglobulin (Ig)G banding. Reproduced courtesy of Professor S. Poser.

in central afferent pathways is due to demyelination; preservation of the response amplitude is typical and reflects relative axonal sparing in MS lesions (Figure 3.11).

Diagnostic criteria

The diagnosis of MS rests on the principle that CNS lesions must be disseminated in space (DIS), i.e. in different areas of the CNS; and disseminated in time (DIT), i.e. at intervals separated by at least 1 month of recovery or an interval in which the dysfunction from a previous attack clearly stabilizes. As the sophistication of MRI has increased, the diagnostic criteria for MS have been repeatedly reviewed and revised. The 'McDonald' diagnostic criteria in use today are named after Professor Ian McDonald, formerly neurologist at the

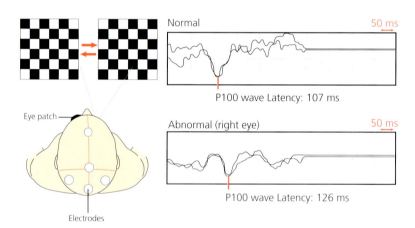

Figure 3.11 Visual evoked potentials (VEPs) are measured by stimulating each eye with an alternating checkerboard pattern. A positive peak at approximately 100 ms (in normal individuals) after stimulation (P100), measured over the visual cortex, is the most common waveform analyzed in VEP studies. Here, the P100 is delayed to 126 ms in the right eye (normal < 108 ms), confirming a 'slowing' of conduction in that optic nerve due to demyelination. Impaired optic nerve conduction determined by VEPs is commonly observed in the absence of a history of visual symptoms or optic neuritis.

Clinical case: a 32-year-old woman presented with a 4-day history of painful lower limb dysesthesias with electrical shock-like sensations in her limbs on neck flexion. MRI of the brain and spine demonstrated a non-enhancing lesion in the cervical spinal cord and two other non-enhancing lesions in her brain in a distribution consistent with demyelination. Her blood tests showed no serological evidence of systemic autoimmunity and aquaporin 4 antibodies were not detected. The CSF did not contain oligoclonal bands.

Further history revealed that the patient had a documented episode of left optic neuritis 16 years ago that had responded to intravenous methylprednisolone.

Discussion: even though the patient does not meet the MRI criteria or the CSF criteria (negative for oligoclonal bands) for MS, her clinical history alone demonstrates dissemination in time and place. Therefore, she has clinically definite MS. The only conundrum here was that she had an 'optico-spinal' presentation and it was therefore important to exclude MS mimics such as neuromyelitis optica.

National Hospital for Neurology and Neurosurgery, London, who initially described the criteria in 2001; they have since been revised in 2005 and 2010. The aims of the latest 2010 revisions were to simplify the MRI criteria for DIS and DIT, and to more clearly define the diagnostic criteria for primary progressive MS (Table 3.5).

Differential diagnosis

It is important to consider and exclude the much rarer alternative causes of inflammatory demyelination within the CNS, such as neuromyelitis optica (NMO) and acute disseminated encephalomyelitis (ADEM), similar yet distinct conditions (Table 3.6). Red flag features that suggest an alternative diagnosis are listed in Table 3.7.

Neuromyelitis optica is a predominantly relapsing inflammatory demyelinating disorder of the CNS that manifests with optic neuritis

43

TABLE 3.5

McDonald (2010) criteria for the diagnosis of multiple sclerosis

Clinical presentation	Additional requirement for diagnosis
≥ 2 attacks; objective clinical evidence of ≥ 2 lesions or objective evidence of 1 lesion with reasonable evidence of a prior attack	None, after other conditions are excluded
≥ 2 attacks; objective clinical evidence of 1 lesion	Dissemination in space (DIS): • ≥ 1 T2 lesion in at least two MS-typical CNS regions*; *or* • Await a further clinical attack implicating a different CNS site
1 attack; objective clinical evidence of ≥ 2 lesions	Dissemination in time (DIT): • Simultaneous asymptomatic gadolinium-enhancing and non-enhancing lesions at any time; *or* • A new T2 and/or gadolinium-enhancing lesion(s) on follow-up MRI irrespective of timing with reference to baseline scan; *or* • Await a second clinical attack
1 attack; objective clinical evidence of 1 lesion (CIS)	Dissemination in space and time For DIS: • ≥ 1 T2 lesion in at least two MS-typical CNS regions*; *or* • Await a second clinical attack implicating a different CNS site For DIT: • Simultaneous asymptomatic gadolinium-enhancing and non-enhancing lesions at any time; *or* • A new T2 and/or gadolinium-enhancing lesion(s) on follow-up MRI irrespective of timing with reference to baseline scan; *or* • Await a second clinical attack

CONTINUED

TABLE 3.5 (CONTINUED)

Clinical presentation	Additional requirement for diagnosis
Insidious neurological progression suggestive of MS	1 year of disease progression plus any two of the following: • Evidence for DIS in the brain based on ≥ 1 T2 lesion(s) in MS-typical regions of the brain* • Evidence for DIS in the spinal cord based on ≥ 2 T2 lesions in the cord • Positive CSF†

*Periventricular, juxtacortical and infratentorial (in the brain) and spinal cord.
†Evidence of oligoclonal bands and/or elevated immunoglobulin G index (see page 41).
CIS, clinically isolated syndrome; CNS, central nervous system;
CSF, cerebrospinal fluid; DIS, disseminated in space; DIT, disseminated in time.
Adapted from Polman CH et al. 2011.

and longitudinally extensive (spanning three or more vertebral segments) transverse myelitis (LETM), although these index events may be separated by years and, in some cases, decades. Distinct clinical imaging (Figures 3.12 and 3.13) and laboratory and pathological features help to distinguish NMO from MS, although the diagnostic criteria remain in a state of flux. The seminal discovery of serum antibodies ('NMO immunoglobulin G') to the water channel aquaporin 4 (AQP-4) in more than 70% of NMO cases suggests a discrete pathogenesis. AQP-4 is primarily expressed on astrocyte foot processes, and recent pathological findings have confirmed that widespread astrocyte destruction precedes inflammatory demyelination in NMO.

Importantly, conventional MS therapies (interferon beta) may exacerbate NMO, and immunosuppression (azathioprine, mycophenolate, rituximab) forms the mainstay of treatment for managing this condition. Early post-marketing data from Japan suggest that fingolimod may also exacerbate NMO. The detection of AQP-4 antibodies in patients with limited disease (either LETM or optic neuritis, but not both), and in patients with a variety of inflammatory brain lesions, has led to the introduction of the term

45

TABLE 3.6

Differential diagnoses of multiple sclerosis

CNS inflammatory demyelination
- Neuromyelitis optica (Devic's syndrome)
- Acute disseminated encephalomyelitis

Other causes of multifocal CNS disease
- Systemic lupus erythematosus (SLE)
- Sjögren's syndrome
- Antiphospholipid antibody syndrome
- Neurosarcoidosis
- Behçet's syndrome
- Susac's syndrome
- CLIPPERS
- CNS histiocytosis
- Cerebral vasculitis (often associated with headache)
- Vitamin B_{12}/folate/copper deficiency (subacute combined degeneration)
- CNS infections (neuroborreliosis, HIV, HTLV-1, tuberculosis)
- Leukodystrophy (especially ALD)

ALD, adrenoleukodystrophy; CLIPPERS, Chronic Lymphocytic Inflammation with Pontine Perivascular Enhancement Responsive to Steroids; CNS, central nervous system; HIV, human immunodeficiency virus; HTLV, human T-lymphotrophic virus.

NMO spectrum disorder. The nosology, pathogenesis, disease course and appropriate treatment trajectory in patients with clinical and radiological features of NMO, but no detectable AQP-4 antibodies, is currently a matter of intense debate.

Acute disseminated encephalomyelitis is predominantly a childhood disease that presents with encephalopathy, which is a rare feature in MS. A history of a preceding systemic infection or immunization

TABLE 3.7

Red flag features that suggest differential diagnoses for multiple sclerosis

- Abrupt onset of neurological symptoms
- Progressive neurological symptoms from onset
- Incomplete recovery from the index episode or initial relapses, with early accruement of disability
- Evidence of involvement of the peripheral nervous system or muscle
- Systemic features such as fever, lung or skin lesions, lymphadenopathy
- Atypical findings on MRI (hemorrhage, leptomeningeal enhancement) or CSF (pleocytosis > 100; protein > 1g)

CSF, cerebrospinal fluid; CNS, central nervous system.

should be sought. The condition is almost exclusively monophasic. High-dose steroids and, rarely, intravenous immunoglobulin/plasma exchange may be required for treatment.

Systemic autoimmunity, including systemic lupus erythematosus (SLE), antiphospholipid antibody syndrome and Sjögren's disease, may present with subacute myelitis or, less commonly, optic neuritis and should be excluded in all patients by thorough history, examination and appropriate serologic testing. Headache, seizures and neuropsychiatric phenomena are atypical in MS; these are more common neurological features of systemic autoimmunity, particularly SLE. A history of sicca symptoms, rash, mouth ulceration, arthralgias, myalgias, Raynaud's phenomenon, alopecia, recurrent miscarriage or venous thrombosis, and the presence of livedo reticularis, lymphadenopathy or arthritis, should especially alert the neurologist to the possibility of these systemic autoimmune disorders.

Sarcoidosis, a granulomatous disease of unknown etiology, may affect the CNS and present with relapsing neurological symptoms that can be

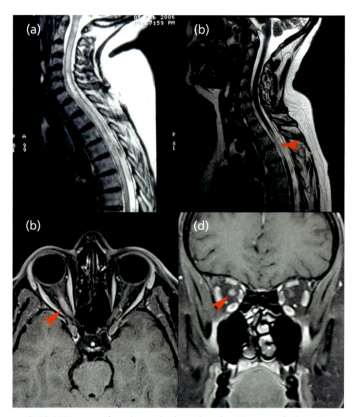

Figure 3.12 MRI scans showing spinal cord and optic nerve lesions in neuromyelitis optica (NMO): (a) T2-weighted imaging, showing prototypic longitudinally extensive holocord inflammation and diffuse cord swelling in acute symptomatic AQP-4-positive NMO relapse. NMO spinal cord lesions may show patchy enhancement and, unlike MS, are usually centrally located and hypointense on T1-weighted sequences; (b) T2-weighted imaging, showing severe atrophy (arrowhead) in a chronic thoracic spinal cord NMO lesion spanning three vertebral segments (T2–T4); (c) axial and (d) coronal contrast-enhanced fat-suppressed T1-weighted imaging, showing acute swelling and enhancement of the right optic nerve (arrowheads) during symptomatic AQP-4-positive NMO relapse with severe right eye visual loss. Optic neuritis in NMO commonly involves a long segment of the optic nerve associated with swelling and enhancement acutely. Bilateral optic nerve involvement and extension posteriorly into the chiasm is common in NMO, but rare in MS. Reproduced with permission from Barnett Y et al. 2014.

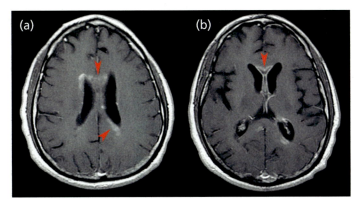

Figure 3.13 MRI scans showing brain lesions in neuromyelitis optica (NMO). Brain lesions occur in more than 60% of patients with NMO, and are commonly located at sites rich in AQP-4, including the brainstem and periependymal regions. Enhancement patterns in acute lesions that are relatively specific for NMO include (a) patchy, 'cloud-like' enhancement (arrowheads) (contrast-enhanced T1-weighted imaging); and (b) 'pencil-thin' ependymal enhancement (arrowhead) (contrast-enhanced T1-weighted imaging). Reproduced with permission from Barnett Y et al. 2014.

mistaken for MS. Afro-Caribbean and northern European (especially Scandinavian) populations are particularly susceptible, and the peak age at disease onset of 20–40 years overlaps with that of MS. Neurosarcoidosis usually occurs in the context of systemic disease, most commonly involving the lymph nodes, lungs or skin (erythema nodosum). In these cases, imaging (chest radiograph, chest CT or whole body 18-fluoro-deoxyglucose positron emission tomography [FDG PET] scan) may be helpful in guiding a biopsy site to establish a tissue diagnosis. Rarely, patients may present with CNS complications of isolated neurosarcoidosis. This entity may be difficult to differentiate from MS on both clinical and radiological grounds. Leptomeningeal enhancement, usually absent in MS, is found in approximately 40% of patients with neurosarcoidosis, and parenchymal lesions may show persistent gadolinium enhancement lasting months or longer (Figure 3.14). Neurosarcoidosis may be steroid-responsive in some patients, in which case the diagnosis only becomes apparent with close clinical and radiological surveillance.

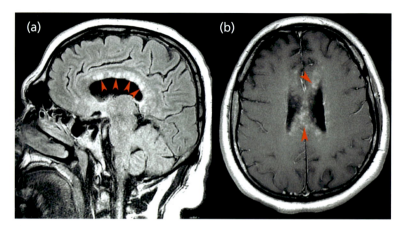

Figure 3.14 MRI scan showing characteristic features of neurosarcoidosis in a 38-year-old man with fluctuating encephalopathy and widespread systemic disease: (a) sagittal fluid-attenuated inversion recovery (FLAIR) imaging, showing multiple lesions in the corpus callosum (arrowheads) that could in isolation be mistaken for MS; (b) axial contrast-enhanced T1-weighted imaging, showing nodular callosal and periependymal enhancement (arrowheads) in the same patient. Images courtesy of Dr Y Barnett.

Rarer inflammatory disorders that can affect the CNS and mimic MS include Behçet's disease, Susac's syndrome, CLIPPERS (Chronic Lymphocytic Inflammation with Pontine Perivascular Enhancement Responsive to Steroids), CNS histiocytosis and cerebral vasculitis.

Prognosis

Whilst it is not always possible to predict the clinical outcome in individual patients, there are some features that may confer either a good or poor prognosis (Table 3.8). Natural history studies have suggested that 10 years from diagnosis, up to 10% of patients have an expanded disability status score (EDSS; see below) greater than 6.5, and up to 40% are unable to work full time. Much of the employment compromise in these patients is due to non-motor symptoms such as cognitive disability, bladder dysfunction and fatigue. In the modern era, these alarming figures may be mitigated by the advent of MRI and the capacity to diagnose and treat MS early in the disease course; the introduction of highly efficacious therapies for relapsing MS; and the

TABLE 3.8

Factors that influence prognosis in multiple sclerosis

Better prognosis	Worse prognosis
Young age of onset	Older age of onset
Female sex	Male sex
Presentation with optic neuritis	'Multifocal' onset
	Motor / cerebellar system affected
Isolated sensory symptom	High relapse rate in first 2–5 years
Full recovery from attack	
Long interval to second relapse	Substantial disability after 5 years
	Large lesion load
No disability after 5 years	Genomic factors (e.g. APOE4 allele indicates more severe disease and faster progression of disability)
Low lesion load	

recognized benefits of multidisciplinary team involvement. The rights of employees with a diagnosis of MS are also now protected, which may enable people with MS to stay in the workplace for longer.

Monitoring disease progression. MS is a chronic condition with an unpredictable course, so it is useful to be able to monitor changes in the level of disability over time.

The Expanded Disability Status Scale provides an amalgamated score that incorporates ambulatory capacity and neurological testing across seven functional domains – visual (optic), brainstem (cranial nerve function including speech and swallowing), pyramidal (motor function), cerebellar (coordination), sensory (touch and pain), bowel and bladder, and cerebral (cognition and mood). Each domain is given a functional system score from 0 (no disability) to 5 or 6 (severe disability). 'Specimen' functional system score definitions can be downloaded at www.neurostatus.net/media/specimen/Definitions_0309_specimen.pdf (last accessed, 28 January 2014).

The total EDSS score ranges from 0 (normal examination) to 10 (death) in 0.5 unit increments (Table 3.9) The EDSS is commonly used

51

TABLE 3.9

Expanded Disability Status Scale

Score	Description
1.0	No disability, minimal signs in one FS
1.5	No disability, minimal signs in more than one FS
2.0	Minimal disability in one FS
2.5	Mild disability in one FS or minimal disability in two FS
3.0	Moderate disability in one FS, or mild disability in three or four FS. No impairment to walking
3.5	Moderate disability in one FS and more than minimal disability in several others. No impairment to walking
4.0	Significant disability but self-sufficient and up and about some 12 hours a day. Able to walk without aid or rest for 500 m
4.5	Significant disability but up and about much of the day, able to work a full day, may otherwise have some limitation of full activity or require minimal assistance. Able to walk without aid or rest for 300 m
5.0	Disability severe enough to impair full daily activities and ability to work a full day without special provisions. Able to walk without aid or rest for 200 m
5.5	Disability severe enough to preclude full daily activities. Able to walk without aid or rest for 100 m
6.0	Requires a walking aid – cane, crutch etc. – to walk about 100 m with or without resting
6.5	Requires two walking aids – a pair of canes, crutches etc. – to walk about 20 m without resting
7.0	Unable to walk beyond approximately 5 m even with aid. Essentially restricted to wheelchair; though wheels self in standard wheelchair and transfers alone. Up and about in wheelchair some 12 hours a day
7.5	Unable to take more than a few steps. Restricted to wheelchair and may need aid in transferring. Can wheel self but cannot carry on in standard wheelchair for a full day and may require a motorized wheelchair

CONTINUED

TABLE 3.9 (CONTINUED)

Score	Description
8.0	Essentially restricted to bed or chair or pushed in wheelchair. May be out of bed itself much of the day. Retains many self-care functions. Generally has effective use of arms
8.5	Essentially restricted to bed much of day. Has some effective use of arms. Retains some self-care functions
9.0	Confined to bed. Can still communicate and eat
9.5	Confined to bed and totally dependent. Unable to communicate effectively or eat/swallow
10	Death

FS, functional system: for specimen FS score definitions, see www.neurostatus.net/media/specimen/Definitions_0309_specimen.pdf, last accessed 12 March 2014.

to assess disability in clinical practice and clinical trials, to gauge how rapidly the disease is progressing and to identify when a patient with MS moves into the secondary progressive phase of disease. In clinical trials, the EDSS is a useful internationally recognized tool for establishing a standard across large groups of patients, enabling comparison of like for like populations. However, the EDSS is an imperfect measure of the impact of disability in MS; it is weighted heavily toward ambulatory capacity, particularly for scores beyond 5.0, and is less affected by important factors such as impaired cognition.

In the later stages of the disease, when disability has progressed, reduced mobility can have significant effects on mortality. It has been established that once a certain level of disability is reached, regardless of the route or time taken to get there, from that point onwards the rate of accumulation of disability is uniformly steady. After EDSS 4.0, there is a steady rate of disability accumulation to reach EDSS 6.0, 8.0 (bedbound) and onwards.

MRI is routinely used to monitor disease activity and progression and response to disease-modifying therapy. MRI may show evidence of subclinical disease activity (gadolinium-enhancing lesions, new or enlarging T2 lesions), progressive loss of brain volume (Figure 3.15) and the accumulation of persistent T1 hypointensities (black holes). MRI findings at presentation can be useful for predicting disease progression. In a 20-year study, lesion volume and its change at earlier time points was found to correlate with the degree of disability. The rate of lesion growth was three times higher in those who developed secondary progressive MS than in those who remained relapsing remitting (Figure 3.16). Rates of whole brain atrophy in the first 1–2 years of the disease have also been shown to predict EDSS scores after 10 years' disease duration.

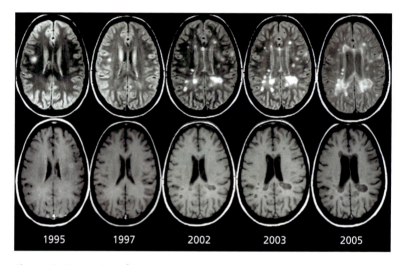

1995 1997 2002 2003 2005

Figure 3.15 A series of MRI scans showing irreversible tissue loss in a patient with relapsing remitting multiple sclerosis (MS) over a 10-year period. While MS is believed to be an inflammatory disease, it clearly has a 'degenerative' component, which becomes more evident with time. Notice both the global volume loss and the enlargement of existing black holes. Reproduced courtesy of Dr Alex Rovira.

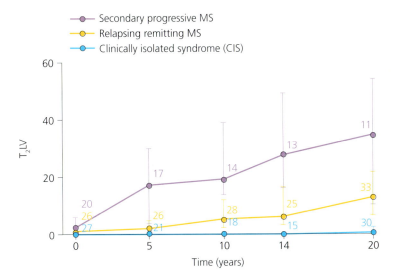

Figure 3.16 Median T2 lesion volume (T$_2$LV) over time. Although there is some overlap in lesion volume at baseline, from 5 years onwards the groups of patients (CIS, relapsing remitting MS, secondary progressive MS) are well distinguished. Patients who developed secondary progressive MS show a greater rate of increase in T2 lesion volume, especially over the first 5 years. Reproduced with permission from Fisniku LK et al. 2008.

Key points – the clinical picture

- The clinical presentation of multiple sclerosis (MS) depends on the location of inflammatory lesions in the central nervous system (CNS). Pathology in the optic nerve, spinal cord and brainstem can result in a broad range of signs and symptoms. However, the majority of deep white matter lesions in the hemispheres are clinically silent.
- People with MS do not always present with the first episode of demyelination. It is therefore important to determine whether the patient has experienced a prior neurological disturbance of any sort (e.g. mild or temporary visual blurring).
- The first presentation due to demyelination within the CNS is termed a clinically isolated syndrome (CIS).
- To diagnose MS, lesions must be shown to be present, separated by time and location.
- The number of asymptomatic demyelinating lesions on MRI at the time of a CIS strongly predicts the likelihood of the patient developing clinically definite MS.
- There are different patterns of MS: relapsing remitting, secondary progressive, primary progressive, progressive relapsing and benign. The subtype of MS will guide prognosis and choice of disease-modifying therapy.
- Rarer alternative causes of inflammatory demyelination within the CNS such as neuromyelitis optica (NMO) and acute disseminated encephalomyelitis (ADEM) should be considered and excluded in the diagnostic work-up of MS.
- Red flag features that suggest an alternative diagnosis include involvement of the peripheral nervous system, atypical MRI findings or systemic features of disease.
- MRI is the most important investigation in the diagnosis and monitoring of MS.
- MS progression can be measured using the expanded disability status score (EDSS) and with MRI.

Key references

Barnett Y, Sutton IJ, Ghadiri M et al. Conventional and advanced imaging in neuromyelitis optica. *AJNR: Am J Neuroradiol* 2014 (10.3174/ajnr. A3592). www.ajnr.org/content/early/2013/06/13/ajnr.A3592.full. pdf, last accessed 12 March 2014.

Degenhardt A, Ramagopalan SV, Scalfari A, Ebers GC. Clinical prognostic factors in multiple sclerosis: a natural history review. *Nat Rev Neurol* 2009;5:672–82.

Fisniku LK, Brex PA, Altmann DR et al. Disability and T2 MRI lesions: a 20-year follow-up of patients with relapse onset of multiple sclerosis. *Brain* 2008;131:808–17.

Kim W, Park MS, Lee SH et al. Characteristic brain magnetic resonance imaging abnormalities in central nervous system aquaporin-4 autoimmunity. *Mult Scler* 2010; 16:1229–36.

Kurtzke JF. Rating neurologic impairment in multiple sclerosis: an expanded disability status scale (EDSS). *Neurology* 1983;33: 1444–52.

Miller DH, Weinshenker BG, Filippi M et al. Differential diagnosis of suspected multiple sclerosis: a consensus approach. *Mult Scler* 2008;14:1157–74.

NICE. Management of multiple sclerosis in primary and secondary care. Clinical Guideline 8. NICE, 2003. http://guidance.nice.org.uk/ CG8, last accessed 12 March 2014.

Papadapoulos MC, Verkman AS. Aquaporin 4 and neuromyelitis optica. *Lancet Neurol* 2012;11: 535–44.

Polman CH, Reingold SC, Banwell B et al. Diagnostic criteria for multiple sclerosis: 2010 revisions to the McDonald criteria. *Ann Neurol* 2011;69:292–302.

Río J, Comabella M, Montalban X. Multiple sclerosis: current treatment algorithms. *Curr Opin Neurol* 2011;24:230–7.

Wakerley B, Nicholas R, Malik O. Multiple sclerosis. *Med Int* 2012;40:523–48.

Treating relapses

A relapse is a period of acute neurological disturbance that lasts for at least 24 hours and is not attributable to other causes such as infection or changes in core temperature.

Corticosteroids are the mainstay of acute treatment for multiple sclerosis (MS) relapses. Evidence suggests that corticosteroids shorten relapse duration but do not alter functional outcome. Corticosteroid therapy is therefore reserved for patients with disabling relapses or patients with an occupational or other need to recover function faster than the natural history of the condition allows.

Corticosteroids have both short- and medium-/long-term risks (Table 4.1), and judicious short-course therapy is therefore essential. Bone loss can occur within weeks of starting continuous oral steroid therapy; calcium/vitamin D supplementation and, in some cases, bisphosphonate therapy should therefore be prescribed for those at risk of fractures and osteoporosis. For patients with a clear history of acid dyspepsia, concurrent proton pump inhibition is also advisable.

TABLE 4.1

Risks associated with corticosteroid use in MS

Short term	Medium and long term
Exacerbation of glycemic control	Hypertension
Delayed wound healing	Lipid disorders
Skin disorders	Osteoporosis
Infections	Weight gain
	Cataracts
	Avascular necrosis of the femoral head

Methylprednisolone. Dosing regimens of 1 g/day for 3 days or 0.5 g/day for 5 days, administered intravenously, are standard. Side effects include facial flushing, palpitations, insomnia and metallic taste. However, oral methylprednisolone, 0.5 g/day for 5 days, has been found to be as effective as intravenous administration and, where this treatment is available, avoids the need for in-patient treatment.

Prednisolone/prednisone is available in a number of oral dosing regimens, starting at 40–60 mg/day, followed by a variable weaning period. However, evidence supporting the use of oral prednisolone/prednisone is limited and there is no indication for prolonged oral steroid therapy following MS relapse. The results of the Optic Neuritis Treatment Trial indicate that administration of moderate-dose oral prednisone, 60 mg/day, to patients with acute optic neuritis actually increases the risk of recurrence. For this reason, high-dose oral or intravenous methylprednisolone is the authors' preferred treatment choice for acute relapse.

Managing symptoms

Neuroinflammation and neurodegeneration culminate in a variety of persistent symptoms that are not necessarily related to acute relapse. The most common are:

- spasticity
- fatigue
- bladder problems
- bowel problems
- pain
- reduction in mobility
- epilepsy and mood disorders.

Changes in 'homeostatic' (normal physiological) function can exacerbate existing MS symptoms. Travel to areas of warm climate, exercise or pyrexia can result in overheating and transient deterioration in neurological function (Uhtoff's phenomenon). Intercurrent infection (bacterial or otherwise) activates inflammatory cytokines, which can result in a 'pseudo-relapse'. It is therefore important to exclude these types of exacerbation, particularly by checking for urinary sepsis, as they can be quickly and completely alleviated with appropriate antimicrobial and antipyretic therapies.

Spasticity is a source of significant discomfort and disability in people with MS. Proactive management in a multidisciplinary setting is needed, with input from neurologists, rehabilitation physicians, physiotherapists and occupational therapists (see Chapter 8).

Oral treatment. Baclofen is the most commonly used first-line antispasticity agent. Second-line pharmacotherapies include tizanidine, gabapentin, dantrolene and benzodiazepines (Table 4.2). These therapies should be started at a low dose and gradually up-titrated to avoid sedation and other side effects.

These classes of drug increase inhibitory influences in the CNS by acting on gamma-aminobutyric acid (GABA) and glycine pathways. They tend to reduce muscle tone and as a consequence can exacerbate or unmask limb weakness. In addition, they may cause sedation and/or worsen speech, swallowing and bladder symptoms, and rarely lead to hepatic dysfunction. Newer antispasticity agents such as gabapentin have a better side-effect profile and are being used increasingly.

Cannabinoids. Recent trials have suggested that cannabinoid-derived compounds may also have a role in this area. These include the oro-mucosally administered nabiximols (Sativex) and the oral medication nabilone. In a proportion of patients with MS, nabiximols, which contains delta-9-tetrahydro-cannabinol (THC) and cannabidiol (CBD) at a 1:1 fixed ratio, has been shown to improve self-reported spasticity scores, sleep disruption and the Barthel Activities of Daily Living index when added to baseline stable therapies such as baclofen or tizanidine. Nabiximols is well tolerated and appears to have minimal psychotropic effects at standard doses (a maximum of 12 sprays in any 24-hour period).

Botulinum toxin type A is a useful therapy for patients with severe focal spasticity. Once injected directly into the affected muscles, botulinum toxin blocks neuromuscular transmission by decreasing acetylcholine release, resulting in temporary reduction of muscle contraction that usually lasts for a few months. Like other antispasticity pharmacotherapies, botulinum toxin should be used in conjunction with physical therapy. The side effects are usually mild and temporary; most commonly, patients report excessive muscle weakness in injected muscles or unexpected patterns of weakness due

TABLE 4.2

Antispasticity agents

	Diazepam	Baclofen	Dantrolene sodium	Tizanidine	Gabapentin
Daily dose	2–15 mg, divided doses	15–100 mg, divided doses	25–400 mg, divided doses	2–36 mg, divided doses	300–3300 mg/day, divided doses
Mode of action	Acts on GABA-mediated inhibitory circuits	Acts as a GABA agonist at spinal level	Acts peripherally on inhibitory circuits	α_2-adrenoreceptor agonist at spinal level	GABA agonist, may inhibit 'new' synapse formation
Common side effects	Drowsiness Confusion Ataxia Paradoxical increase in aggression Dependency	Sedation Drowsiness Nausea Lassitude Dizziness Ataxia Depression Tremor	Drowsiness Dizziness Fatigue Diarrhea Nausea Headache Liver dysfunction	Dry mouth Somnolence Asthenia Dizziness Headache	Sedation Confusion Ataxia Fatigue

GABA, gamma-aminobutyric acid.

61

to inadvertent injection of incorrect muscle groups. Increasing 'selectivity' using electromyography (EMG)-guided injections is becoming a highly specialized field. Systemic side effects are rare.

More radical treatments. In intractable spasticity, particularly affecting the lower limbs, more radical approaches may be required. These include invasive techniques such as injection of drugs directly into the spinal space (intrathecal baclofen pumps) or medical/surgical rhizotomy (selective destruction of relevant spinal nerve roots).

Balcofen pumps are a useful way of providing continuous control of severe chronic spasticity. Patients receiving high levels of oral antispasticity medications may feel that a continuous infusion is preferable to multiple tablets, especially if swallowing has been affected or if systemic side effects are unacceptable.

Following a comprehensive assessment of spasticity, a trial dose of intrathecal baclofen, 50–100 µg, is usually given before insertion of a permanent baclofen pump. Repeated assessments should be performed over the next 4–8 hours to determine whether intrathecal baclofen results in objective improvement in the patient's spasticity.

Baclofen pumps are inserted under general anesthesia beneath the abdominal muscles. Once the pump is inserted, doses are slowly titrated up until a therapeutic response is obtained. Potential adverse effects include:

- lack of efficacy
- leakage from the system leading to under-dosing
- pooling of baclofen with local irritant effects
- infection.

Baclofen pumps require regular follow-up and assessment in a subspecialist clinic.

Fatigue affects at least 80% of people with MS, with most reporting it as one of their most disabling symptoms. The physiological basis for fatigue is yet to be fully established. At the cellular level, fatigue may result from the need for additional energy to transmit impulses along demyelinated axons, without the benefit of saltatory conduction. Fatigue is a common symptom during relapse, but may follow a course independent of clinical and imaging markers or disease activity.

Clinical case: a 39-year-old woman with a 20-year history of progressive MS and very limited mobility (EDSS 6.5) had profound spasticity. She was unable to tolerate oral baclofen, tizanidine, dantrolene, clonazepam or even cannabinoids. Severe extensor and adductor spasms in her lower limbs prevented adequate provision of care at home, which resulted in worsening pain and impeded safe intermittent bladder catheterization. Following multidisciplinary assessment, a trial of intrathecal baclofen was advised with a view to insertion of a baclofen pump.

Discussion: in treatment-refractory spasticity, intrathecal baclofen has many advantages. The direct infusion of baclofen into the thecal sac allows smaller doses to be used with fewer systemic side effects. Programmable pumps permit exact dose titration that can be varied throughout the day, providing the patient with the capacity to control their own spasticity more precisely.

Fatigue may also be the presenting feature of a mood disorder (depression), which should be sought and treated proactively.

A better understanding of the pathophysiological mechanisms that underlie fatigue may yield novel approaches to treatment. Clearly defining and quantifying MS-related fatigue (e.g. with the MS Fatigue Severity Score) will help standardize the results of future clinical trials.

Non-pharmacological approaches. Cognitive behavioral therapy may be employed as part of a multidisciplinary approach. For example, the 'Fatigue: Applying Cognitive behavioral and Energy effectiveness Techniques to lifeStyle (FACETS)' program has shown some benefit in patients with MS. Graduated exercise programs and cardiovascular conditioning may also be helpful.

Pharmacological approaches. Amantadine, 100 mg twice daily, may exert a modest effect in some patients but solid clinical trial data are lacking; and anticholinergic side effects limit its utility in patients with MS. Modafinil, 200–400 mg daily, promotes wakefulness through interaction with a variety of neurotransmitters, though its

63

precise mechanism of action is unknown. Use in MS is limited by lack of reimbursement for this indication in some countries and side effects, which may include irritability, headaches and insomnia.

Bladder and bowel problems may occur in the context of an MS relapse, and thus management of the relapse can sometimes alleviate associated sphincter dysfunction in the short term. However, bowel and particularly bladder symptoms (frequency, urgency, urge incontinence) can become established and chronic in MS. Multidisciplinary treatment involving neurologists, primary care providers, urologists, gastroenterologists and continence advisors/ nurses is often required.

Bladder problems occur in more than 70% of people with MS. In early MS, detrusor hyperactivity (primarily due to disruption of descending inhibitory inputs from the spinal cord) is the most common etiology. Investigation of bladder dysfunction in MS includes:

- exclusion of (coexistent) urinary tract infection
- measurement of the post-void residual volume (see below)
- urodynamic studies.

The key to management is to first establish whether bladder emptying is satisfactory. In patients with a significant post-voiding residual volume of urine (more than 100 mL), intermittent self-catheterization is the primary treatment strategy (Figure 4.1). Usually, the patient is taught this technique, but physical issues such as poor upper limb function (strength or coordination) or significant lower limb spasticity (adductor spasms) may prevent this approach. In these circumstances, insertion of an indwelling catheter (urethral or preferably suprapubic) may be necessary. All patients should be advised to maintain adequate fluid intake.

Patients with symptomatic detrusor activity and post-voiding residual urinary volumes of less than 100 mL are initially treated with bladder antispasmodics, including:

- oxybutynin, 5–15 mg daily (in divided doses)
- tolterodine, 2–4 mg daily (in divided doses)
- solifenacin, 5 mg daily.

(a)

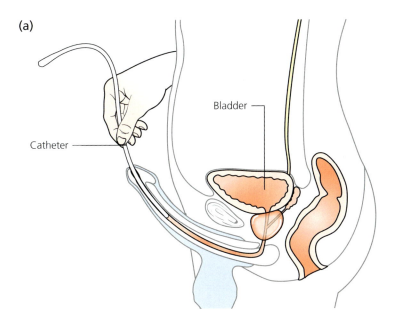

(b)

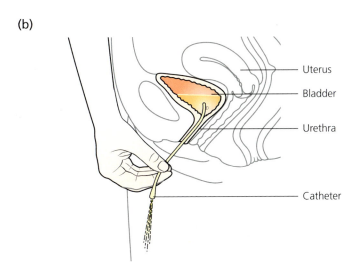

Figure 4.1 Self-catheterization in (a) men and (b) women. Reproduced with permission from Diane K Newman.

The use of these drugs is limited by anticholinergic side effects (e.g. dry mouth and constipation), and if they lead to an increase in the urinary residual volume their use should be reconsidered. However, they may be used in combination with intermittent self-catheterization in patients with high urinary residual volumes and symptomatic detrusor overactivity. They may also be used as required in patients with mild urinary frequency and urgency. Desmopressin, 10–20 µg at night, is helpful in younger patients with nocturnal frequency and incontinence. Care should be taken to avoid fluid overload.

A specialist urologic review should be sought for all patients who do not respond to anticholinergic therapies. Formal urodynamic studies may indicate more complex bladder dysfunction. If urgency and frequency are refractory to treatment, with a low residual of urine, then botulinum toxin A injections into the detrusor muscle via a cystoscope can be very successful (Figure 4.2). Botulinum toxin inhibits neurotransmitter release and reversibly decreases muscle contractility. Regeneration takes place within 5–9 months, so repeated

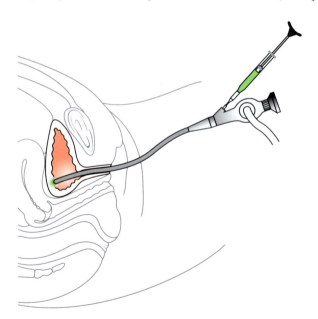

Figure 4.2 Botulinum toxin A is injected via a cystoscope directly into the detrusor muscle.

injections may be necessary. The most important potential adverse effects are detrusor hypotonia and urinary retention.

Occasionally, surgical procedures such as suprapubic catheterization can optimize management (see *Fast Facts: Bladder Disorders*).

Bowel management. The mainstay of treatment is dietary manipulation (e.g. high fiber for constipation) and adequate hydration. Some patients with refractory constipation require regular enemas and laxatives (e.g. senna, lactulose). Diarrhea is a less frequent problem, which may require loperamide or rarely codeine-based compounds; however, care should be taken to exclude 'overflow' diarrhea associated with constipation. Occasionally, 'bacterial overgrowth' syndromes can be an issue, but these are easily diagnosed and treated in conjunction with gastroenterologists. Very rarely, intractable bowel incontinence causing profound social and physical impairment may necessitate colostomy.

Pain is a common accompaniment of MS. It can be divided into acute and chronic pain.

Acute pain

Paroxysmal pain syndromes. Trigeminal neuralgia is a common acute presentation in MS and may be clinically indistinguishable from the idiopathic counterpart. It is usually attributable to a small focus of inflammatory demyelination at the root entry zone of the ipsilateral fifth nerve in the brainstem. Trigeminal neuralgia in MS is usually sensitive to carbamazapine; second-line agents include gabapentin, pregabalin, lamotrigine and baclofen. Tricyclic antidepressants such as amitryptiline and nortryptiline may also be helpful. Rarely, trigeminal neuralgia becomes persistent or recurrent in MS and, if refractory to medical therapy, should prompt neurosurgical review for consideration of local ablative treatments.

Tonic spasms, which can be severe and debilitating, occasionally occur in patients with cervical spinal cord or lower medullary inflammatory demyelination. Ephaptic transmission, 'cross-talk' between hyperexcitable denuded axons within the acute MS lesion, may explain this phenomenon. This symptom is more common in patients with neuromyelitis optica than MS. L'hermitte's phenomenon is an electrical shock-like sensation along the spine and/or limbs associated with neck flexion, which may occasionally be painful and is thought to have a similar pathophysiology. Both conditions usually respond rapidly to the same array of medical therapies used for trigeminal neuralgia, specifically carbamazepine.

Other neuropathic pain syndromes. Acute burning/dysesthetic (spinothalamic) pain occasionally accompanies MS relapse. This pain may have a radicular distribution, but is commonly more diffuse and usually involves the lower limbs. Both anticonvulsant and tricyclic antidepressant therapies may be efficacious in this setting. Newer antidepressants such as the serotonin-norepinephrine reuptake inhibitor (SNRI) duloxetine may be particularly helpful for this indication. All these drugs reduce 'central' transmission of pain impulses either by blocking ion channels (lamotrigine, carbamazepine), increasing inhibitory effects on pain pathways (gabapentin, pregabalin) or altering neurotransmitter balance in favor of pain suppression (amitryptiline, nortryptiline, duloxetine).

Inflammatory pain. The acute inflammation associated with demyelination may give rise to pain. For example, acute retrobulbar optic neuritis can be very uncomfortable, particularly with ocular movement, and responds promptly to steroids administered for the acute relapse.

Migrainous pain. For reasons that are unclear, migraine is more common in patients with MS than in the general population. Some clinicians speculate that this may be due to altered brainstem function in patients with MS, particularly those with lesions in the periaqueductal gray matter of the midbrain. Migraine in patients with MS can be treated with traditional antimigraine drugs such as acetylsalicylic acid (ASA; aspirin), non-steroidal anti-inflammatory drugs (NSAIDs), triptans and, if the symptoms are recurrent, migraine preventive therapies.

Chronic pain. Some of the pain syndromes listed above can become chronic, and a similar approach is used in terms of pharmacological interventions depending on the type of pain (see *Fast Facts: Chronic and Cancer Pain*). Cannabinoids are an adjunct to traditional pain modulators in these circumstances.

Multidisciplinary management with pain specialists who use non-pharmacological techniques can be very helpful. These include psychological therapies, acupuncture and transcutaneous nerve stimulation (TENS). Rare use of stereotactic neurosurgical techniques, whereby stimulating electrodes are placed in strategic areas in the pain pathway (thalamus, periaqueductal gray matter etc.), are being trialled with some success. These techniques are promising but await formal approvals.

Mobility. Gait disturbance affects 80% of people with MS within 10–15 years of diagnosis, and many will need assistance to maintain their mobility. Losing the ability to walk is distressing, and an important aspect of management is the provision of walking aids and appropriate physical therapy to maintain independent mobility. It may be difficult to predict the degree of recovery from acute spinal relapses that impair mobility. Gait disturbance is a dominant feature in progressive forms of MS, reflected in the Kurtzke EDSS rating scale in which limitation of mobility becomes the defining characteristic from EDSS 3.5–7.0 (see Table 3.9, page 52).

People with MS are particularly vulnerable to falling (Table 4.3). Falls can shorten time to wheelchair dependence. Mobility assistance will help to:
- maintain independence
- reduce fatigue
- allow specific activities to continue.

Physical therapy/rehabilitation can improve muscle weakness, spasticity and general wellbeing, particularly in the context of

TABLE 4.3

Factors that increase the risk of falling

• Loss of balance	• Fear of falling
• Weakness	• Spasticity and tremor
• Fatigue	• Visual impairment
• Cognitive impairment	

deconditioning associated with relapses or intercurrent illness. A multidisciplinary approach is especially important in addressing mobility, spasticity, pain control and incontinence. Appropriate adaptations to the home environment in the later stages of MS can maximize function and independent living (Table 4.4).

Pharmacological treatment. The first drug to improve walking in MS was approved in the USA in 2010. Prolonged-release fampridine, a formulation of 4-aminopyridine, is an orally administered potassium-channel blocker that improves walking in some patients with MS. In Europe, it is licensed for patients with an EDSS of 4.0–7.0. Responders (fewer than half of patients in clinical trials) taking a dose of 10 mg twice daily can be identified within the first 4 weeks of treatment; walking speed, as determined by a 25-foot timed walk, improves by an average of 25% in this group. Fampridine is generally well tolerated but side effects can include neuropathic pain, vertigo and, rarely, seizures. A history of seizures is a contraindication to initiating fampridine.

Walking aids. Walking sticks, crutches and wheelchairs are the traditional aids. However, in select individuals ankle foot orthoses (fixed or dynamic splints, Dictus band) can physically correct foot

TABLE 4.4

Home adaptations to maximize function and independent living

Location	Adaptation
Outside	Handrails/ramps for aid of access
Hallway/stairs	Handrails/stairlift
Bathroom	Handrails to aid getting in and out of the bath/toilet; adaptor seat
	Wet room (more easily accessible than a bath)
Kitchen	Bright colors to assist the visually impaired
	Grabbing tools to aid reaching
	Adapted utensils and cutlery
Bedroom	Hoists/ commodes/air mattresses

drop; and functional electrical stimulation has an increasing role in gait maintenance (Figure 4.3).

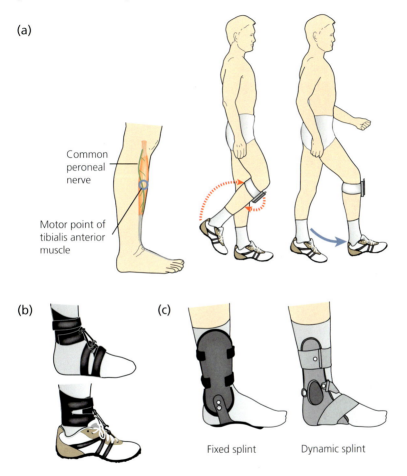

(a)

Common peroneal nerve

Motor point of tibialis anterior muscle

(b)

(c)

Fixed splint   Dynamic splint

Figure 4.3 (a) Functional electrical stimulation: as the heel is raised, a sensor in the shoe signals a microprocessor, which sends an electrical pulse to the common peroneal nerve and the motor point of the tibialis anterior muscle, dorsiflexing the foot and allowing the patient to swing the foot through and walk smoothly. (b) Dictus bands use a recoil and stretch action with a latex elastic band and hook that helps raise the foot after toe-off and reduces the risk of tripping (indoor and outdoor versions shown). (c) Ankle orthotic devices promote dorsiflexion and stability in the leg.

Epilepsy. Seizures were considered rare in demyelinating conditions, which were thought to predominantly involve the white matter. Recent neuropathological studies indicate that gray matter involvement may be extensive in MS, even in early disease (Chapter 2); a higher incidence of cortical/juxtacortical lesions in patients with seizures implicates gray matter disease as the likely substrate for seizures in MS. Partial seizures are usually readily controlled with anticonvulsants such as lamotrigine, levetiracetam, carbamazepine, sodium valproate and topiramate (written in the authors' preferred order) (also see *Fast Facts: Epilepsy*).

Seizures must be differentiated from paroxysmal movement disorders such as tonic spasms, kinesogenic choreoathetosis and some dystonias. The pathophysiology of these conditions is distinct from seizures; for example, aberrant (ephaptic) transmission of nerve impulses has been implicated in tonic spasms. Unlike seizures, they do not impair consciousness, may be painful and often have clear triggers such as changes in position. Careful history taking and, in more complex cases, electrophysiological studies, will help to clarify the diagnosis. Both seizures and paroxysmal symptoms may respond rapidly to anticonvulsant therapy, but a diagnosis of epilepsy can have profound effects on the social/employment status of the patient. In the UK, the patient will be prohibited from driving for 12 months after a single seizure.

Mood disorders, particularly depression, are extremely common in MS. Some studies estimate rates as high as 40%. A concurrent mood disorder may have a profound effect on both physical and cognitive functioning in patients with MS and must be sought and treated aggressively with a program of behavioral therapy, pharmacotherapy and physical exercise. Also see *Fast Facts: Depression*.

Key points – treatment of relapses and symptoms

- Disabling multiple sclerosis (MS) relapses should be treated with high-dose (500–1000 mg/day) short-course (3–5 days) intravenous or oral methylprednisolone.
- Corticosteroid therapy hastens recovery from acute relapse but may not affect ultimate function. There is no indication for prolonged oral steroid therapy following MS relapse.
- Moderate dose (60 mg/day) oral corticosteroid therapy for optic neuritis may increase the risk of recurrence and should be avoided.
- MS symptoms including pain, spasticity and sphincter dysfunction are a source of significant disability and should be treated proactively.
- Spasticity may be severe and is managed in most patients with a combination of physical therapy and oral medication. In severe focal spasticity, botulinum toxin injections have a role.
- Bladder dysfunction commonly manifests with urinary frequency, urgency and urge incontinence and is ameliorated with anticholinergic therapy in most patients with low urinary residual volumes (< 100 mL).
- Intermittent self-catheterization should be considered in patients with significant urinary retention (urinary residual volume > 100 mL), and formal urodynamic studies may be indicated to exclude complex bladder dysfunction.
- Pain in MS most commonly has a neuropathic origin and responds to anticonvulsant therapy or antidepressant (tricyclic or serotonin-norepinephrine reuptake inhibitor) therapy.
- Impaired mobility is a dominant feature of progressive MS, and function should be optimized through multidisciplinary care, provision of appropriate walking aids and, in selected cases, symptomatic treatment with fampridine.
- Depression complicates the course of MS in up to 40% of patients and should be proactively managed with a program of behavioral therapy, pharmacotherapy and physical exercise.

Key references

Ben Smail D, Peskine A, Roche N et al. Intrathecal baclofen for treatment of spasticity of multiple sclerosis patients. *Mult Scler* 2006;12:101–3.

Bible E. Pain: Comorbidity of neuropathic pain and migraine in patients with multiple sclerosis. *Nat Rev Neurol* 2013;9:544

Burton JM, O'Connor PW, Hohol M, Bevene J. Oral versus intravenous steroids for treatment of relapses in multiple sclerosis. *Cochrane Database Syst Rev* 2012;12:CD006921.

de Sa JC, Airas L, Bartholome E et al. Symptomatic therapy in multiple sclerosis: a review for a multimodal approach in clinical practice. *Ther Adv Neurol Disord* 2011;4:139–68.

Gal RL, Vedula SS, Beck R. Corticosteroids for treating optic neuritis. *Cochrane Database Syst Rev* 2012;4:CD001430.

Koch M, Uyttenboogaart M, Polman S, De Keyser J. Seizures in multiple sclerosis. *Epilepsia* 2008;49:948–53.

Krupp LB, LaRocca NG, Muir-Nash J, Steinberg AD. *Arch Neurol* 1989;46:1121–3.

Martyn CN, Illis LS, Thom J. Nabilone in the treatment of multiple sclerosis. *Lancet* 1995;345:579.

Moisset X, Ouchchane L, Guy N et al. Migraine headaches and pain with neuropathic characteristics: comorbid conditions in patients with multiple sclerosis. *Pain* 2013;154: 2691–9.

NHS (England). Clinical Commissioning Policy Document: Fampridine for Multiple Sclerosis. NHS England, April 2013. www.england.nhs.uk/wp-content/uploads/2013/04/d04-ps-d.pdf

Pucci E, Tato PB, D'Amico R et al. Amantadine for fatigue in multiple sclerosis. *Cochrane Database Syst Rev* 2009;CD002818.

Thomas S, Thomas PW, Kersten P et al. A pragmatic parallel arm multi-centre randomised controlled trial to assess the effectiveness and cost-effectiveness of a group-based fatigue management programme (FACETS) for people with multiple sclerosis. *J Neurol Neurosurg Psychiatry* 2013;84:1092–9.

Thompson AJ, Toosy AT, Ciccarelli O. Pharmacological management of symptoms in multiple sclerosis: current approaches and future directions. *Lancet Neurol* 2010;9:1182–99.

Zajicek JP, Ingram WM, Vickery J et al. Patient-orientated longitudinal study of multiple sclerosis in south west England (The South West Impact of Multiple Sclerosis Project, SWIMS) 1: protocol and baseline characteristics of cohort. *BMC Neurol* 2010;10:88.

What is the benefit of treatment?

In general, disease-modifying therapies (DMTs) are used in ambulatory patients with relapsing remitting multiple sclerosis (MS). There is less evidence of benefit in patients with progressive forms of the disease. This may in part reflect the fact that most clinical trials in MS, in which relapse rate and severity are important endpoints, do not enrol patients with progressive disease.

In patients with relapsing disease, existing therapies reduce the rate of relapse and slow the rate of lesion accumulation on MRI, but neither of these endpoints has a clear correlation with disability, and no treatments have been shown to reverse or slow the progression of MS over the longer term. It is important to consider this when initiating treatment, and to be realistic about what each treatment can offer.

Conversely, progression of disability may occur over decades and the true efficacy of existing, newer generation treatments may not yet be apparent.

In the early 1990s, the first clinical trials of immunomodulation produced statistically significant results. Several DMTs are now available:

- interferon beta-1a/b
- glatiramer acetate
- natalizumab
- fingolimod
- teriflunomide
- dimethyl fumarate.

When to start disease-modifying treatment

An initial consideration in the management of MS is when to start treatment and which treatment to choose. Patients with active relapsing disease should generally be treated, and an increasing body of evidence suggests that early therapy has advantages over delayed treatment (Figure 5.1). It is also possible to identify people with

75

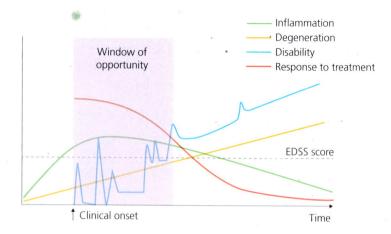

Inflammation
Degeneration
Disability
Response to treatment

Window of opportunity

EDSS score

↑ Clinical onset   Time

Figure 5.1 Window of opportunity for disease-modifying treatment. Current immune-directed disease-modifying treatments (DMTs) target the early inflammatory phase of relapsing MS. With longer disease duration, inflammation recruited from the systemic circulation decreases, and the exhaustion of neuroaxonal reserves manifests with gradually worsening disability. At present, there is no effective therapy in this phase of the disease. Although the relationship between neuroinflammation and neurodegeneration is not well understood, treatment of MS in the early 'window of opportunity' may prevent or delay the time to secondary progression.

clinically isolated syndromes (CIS) who are at greater risk of developing clinically definite MS (see Chapter 3) and may benefit from early initiation of first-line therapies.

Conventional therapy

The conventional first-line therapies in MS are termed 'immunomodulatory' therapies. Interferon beta-1a and -1b modulate the activity of B and T cells. Glatiramer acetate does not have an established mode of action but is thought to act as a 'decoy' that sequesters autoreactive T lymphocytes in the periphery, thus ameliorating immune activation in the central nervous system (CNS).

   Both treatments have been shown, in multiple clinical trials, to reduce relapse rates by 33–38% over a 2-year period, and in most

Clinical case: a 28-year-old man with an established diagnosis of MS presented with three relapses (one brainstem, two optic neuritis) over the previous 3 years. He required intravenous methylprednisolone therapy on two occasions, both with remission to baseline function. His current EDSS was 3.0. Significant background history included inflammatory bowel disease, flares of which were managed with short courses of oral corticosteroids. Brain MRI had not demonstrated a significant change in the total T2 lesion load over 3 years or evidence of active disease (gadolinium-enhancing lesions). His primary care physician specifically asked about new therapeutic opportunities.

Discussion: this patient has experienced annual relapses, including a brainstem attack, and required intravenous steroids on two occasions. Although his brain has shown no evidence of disease activity by way of T2 lesion accumulation or gadolinium enhancement, he clearly requires disease-modifying treatment. Therapy with a conventional first-line agent (interferon beta, glatiramer acetate) or a newer oral agent (fingolimod, dimethyl fumarate or teriflunomide in countries where these therapies are available and have a first-line indication) would be appropriate options. Discussion regarding the relative advantages and disadvantages of each therapy in the context of the patient's medical history and lifestyle will determine the specific treatment choice.

countries are licensed for the treatment of patients with relapsing MS who have experienced two or more clinically significant relapses over the last 2 years. In people with CIS, there is robust evidence that these treatments delay the second clinical attack and therefore the diagnosis of clinically definite MS (CDMS).

Compared with delayed treatment, initiation of conventional DMTs in patients with CIS can delay the diagnosis of CDMS by up to 12 months and reduce disability progression over 2–3 years. However, longer-term studies suggest that DMTs may not significantly alter the

Clinical case: a 54-year-old man with a 7-year history of relapsing remitting MS, but relapse free for 5 years on interferon, presented with a significant spinal cord relapse necessitating admission to hospital for 4 weeks. He also had a history of ischemic heart disease and his ECG showed second degree heart block. He was treated with intravenous methylprednisolone and began to improve. An assay for interferon beta-neutralizing antibodies was strongly positive. Brain and spine MRI showed no gadolinium-enhancing lesions or significant increase in T2 lesion load.

Discussion: the patient suffered a severe attack in the presence of neutralizing antibodies to interferon beta, which probably abrogated the effectiveness of this therapy. An alternative DMT should be considered. Fingolimod is contraindicated by the presence of second degree heart block. The severity of the spinal attack justifies escalating therapy to either natalizumab or dimethyl fumarate. The indications for natalizumab vary from country to country: in the UK and Europe, this case would not meet the requisite radiological criteria for highly active relapsing remitting MS. Similarly, at the time of publication dimethyl fumarate is not available in all countries. In this context, reasonable therapeutic avenues to pursue would be glatiramer acetate or teriflunomide.

patient's ultimate disability. In CIS, brain MRI stratifies the risk of developing CDMS: in patients with abnormal imaging consistent with demyelination, the risk approximates 90% over 15 years. In those with a greater risk of CDMS, there may be an argument for initiating DMTs; the decision must be tailored to the individual on the basis of a risk-benefit discussion. Meanwhile, clinicians, health funding authorities and health economists continue to debate the role of these therapies in patients with CIS in difficult economic times.

Injection issues. The mode and frequency of therapy may affect the treatment decision. Interferons are injected intramuscularly (weekly) or subcutaneously (every other day or three times per week), and glatiramer acetate subcutaneously (daily) (Table 5.1). Rarely, patients have 'needle phobia' and will not contemplate injectable therapy. Despite the lack of long-term safety data in MS populations, they may prefer to consider first-line oral medication if available for this indication. Subcutaneous injectable therapies may be preferable for some patients but this must be balanced with the inconvenience of more frequent dosing. Injection site reactions (redness, swelling) are common with all subcutaneously injected DMTs (Figure 5.2), but generally improve with time. Injection site reactions are less common in patients treated with intramuscular weekly interferon beta-1a (Avonex). Long-term subcutaneous injections may be complicated by lipoatrophy, which is of cosmetic significance in some patients.

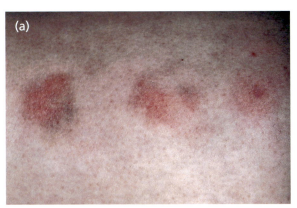

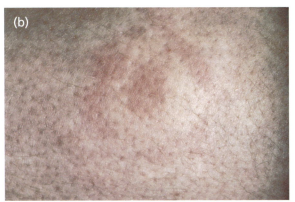

Figure 5.2 Skin reactions to subcutaneous injection of (a) interferon and (b) glatiramer acetate.

TABLE 5.1

Conventional disease-modifying therapy

Drug	Dose/administration	Frequency	Side effects	Comments
Interferon beta-1a (Avonex)	30 μg i.m.	Weekly	Common: flu-like symptoms, mood changes, insomnia Rare: injection site reactions, hepatic dysfunction, alopecia, bone marrow dysfunction	Neutralizing antibodies rare
Interferon beta-1a (Rebif)	22 μg s.c.* 44 μg s.c.	3 x per week 3 x per week	Common: flu-like symptoms, injection site reactions, mood changes, insomnia Rare: bone marrow and hepatic dysfunction, alopecia	'Recrudescence' of side effects can be a sign of neutralizing antibodies
Interferon beta-1b (Betaseron/ Betaferon or Extavia)	250 μg s.c.	Alternate days	Common: flu-like symptoms, injection site reactions, mood changes, insomnia Rare: bone marrow and hepatic dysfunction, alopecia	'Recrudescence' of side effects can be a sign of neutralizing antibodies
Glatiramer acetate (Copaxone)	20 mg s.c.	Daily	Common: injection site reactions Rare: immediate post-injection hypersensitivity reactions	Effective use when interferon neutralizing antibodies are present

*22 μg dose not marketed in all countries.
i.m., intramuscular; s.c., subcutaneous.

Dosage, route of administration and common side effects of the injectable therapies are shown in Table 5.1.

Significant flu-like symptoms are experienced by approximately 50% of patients commencing interferon beta therapy. These can be prevented or alleviated with paracetamol (acetaminophen)/non-steroidal anti-inflammatory drugs (NSAIDs) on the day of injection in most patients. For weekly intramuscular therapy, patients may choose to inject on a day when they have few work or social engagements (commonly at the weekend). It is important to inform patients of the potential side effects so that they can plan for when they need to rest or take prophylactic pain relief. Rarer side effects of interferon beta therapy include mood disorders, alopecia and bone marrow/hepatic dysfunction (which requires regular blood monitoring, as discussed below).

Monitoring. When interferon therapies are initiated, the following blood tests are important:
• full blood count (FBC)
• liver function tests (LFT)
• urea and electrolytes
• protein electrophoresis.

The FBC and LFT should be repeated at 1 month, 3 months and every 6 months thereafter. Liver function abnormalities are most common, and if mild should be observed initially. If there is ongoing and significant liver function test derangement, the interferon dose should be reduced and cessation of treatment considered. This decision is best made by the prescribing clinician.

Rarely, patients with a monoclonal gammopathy who are given interferon therapy can develop a potentially fatal systemic capillary leak syndrome.

Up to 35% of patients taking interferon therapy produce neutralizing antibodies against the drug after 2 years of treatment. These can reduce the efficacy of the treatment and are an indication to consider alternative treatment options.

When to stop conventional treatment. The indications for ceasing first-line treatment are shown in Table 5.2.

TABLE 5.2

Indications for stopping conventional disease-modifying treatment

- Frequent relapses (which are an indication to escalate to second-line therapy)
- Continued decline without any objective evidence of clear relapse (an indication of the progressive phase of the disease, for which no beneficial DMT is currently available)
- Detection of neutralizing antibodies in patients treated with interferon beta
- Intolerable side effects (e.g. persistent flu-like symptoms, injection site problems)

New generation therapies

Intravenous therapy. Natalizumab is a humanized monoclonal antibody against the cell adhesion molecule α4-integrin. It binds to the α4 subunit of the α4β1-integrin and prevents leukocyte adhesion to endothelial vascular cell adhesion molecule-1, thus preventing the migration of immune cells into the CNS (Figure 5.3). Initially licensed

(a)   (b)

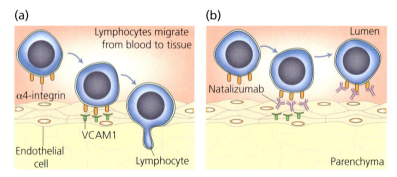

Figure 5.3 (a) The binding of α4-integrin to vascular cell adhesion molecule-1 (VCAM1) on inflamed brain endothelium allows the migration of leukocytes (immune cells) into the central nervous system. (b) By binding to the α4 subunit of the α4β1-integrin, natalizumab prevents leukocyte adhesion to endothelial VCAM1, thereby diminishing the capacity of the adaptive immune response to augment focal CNS inflammation.

Clinical case: a 26-year-old woman developed diplopia, dysarthria and ataxia 6 weeks after the delivery of her first child. Brain MRI showed established T2 lesions and four enhancing lesions, including the presumed symptomatic lesion in the pons. She was treated with intravenous methylprednisolone, prompting an incomplete recovery over several weeks, and she continued to breastfeed her child. Two months later she had a significant spinal cord relapse with a marked spastic paraparesis that required further intravenous methylprednisolone treatment. Although she had a residual gait disturbance, lower limb weakness and spasticity, she was reluctant to start DMT, and continued to breastfeed, against the advice of her neurologist. A further 3 months later she developed severe left optic neuritis; a third course of intravenous methylprednisolone was administered and her vision recovered to 6/9 (20/30) over 6 weeks with persistently abnormal color perception and early pallor of the left optic disc. Brain MRI showed a significant increase in her T2 lesion load and four further enhancing lesions.

Discussion: this patient had highly active (rapidly evolving) relapsing MS with marked MRI activity and three disabling relapses within 9 months. An aggressive treatment approach was warranted and natalizumab therapy was commenced following discussion of the pertinent benefits and risks of this treatment. Her condition stabilized and further recovery from the previous spinal and ocular relapses was evident at review 3 months later.

in the USA in 2004, it was the first therapy of this type for MS and seen as a breakthrough in treatment.

In Europe and the UK, natalizumab is indicated for highly active relapsing remitting MS, usually with both clinically significant relapses *and* markers of radiological activity on a recent MRI scan, such as gadolinium-enhancing lesions or a significant increase in T2 lesion load. The indication in the USA and Australia is broader, but in practice it is predominantly used in the same patient group. Natalizumab has been shown to reduce the annualized relapse rate by

68% and the risk of disability progression sustained for 24 weeks versus placebo by 54%. Given as a monthly infusion of 300 mg (Table 5.3), natalizumab potently reduces inflammatory demyelination and has transformed the management of patients with rapidly evolving disease. Unfortunately, restricted lymphocyte trafficking into the CNS also reduces normal immune surveillance of the brain and contributes to a risk of progressive multifocal leukoencephalopathy (PML), a potentially fatal condition that is due to reactivation of the JC virus (Figure 5.4). There are risk stratification tools that estimate PML risk based on previous exposure to immunosuppressive therapies (such as azathioprine), duration of treatment with natalizumab and serological evidence of previous exposure to the causative JC virus (Figure 5.5).

However, there is no substitute for scrupulous clinical and radiological monitoring of patients. In patients with positive serum assays for JC virus antibody who are maintained on natalizumab, brain MRI should be performed at least 6 monthly (see Figure 5.4). In patients who cease natalizumab on the basis of increased risk of PML (see Figure 5.5), the therapeutic options are limited, as de-escalating therapy may result in a return of MS disease activity. Alemtuzumab, another highly efficacious treatment (see Chapter 6), may be an appropriate agent in such patients in the future. Administration and monitoring of natalizumab therapy is largely restricted to specialist centers and clinicians experienced specifically in the management of MS.

Oral therapy

Fingolimod was the first oral agent to be licensed for relapsing forms of MS. In the USA and Australia it is used as first-line therapy, but is also a second-line treatment for people whose MS remains active despite treatment with conventional DMT. Fingolimod is a novel small molecule modulator of the sphingosine 1-phosphate (S1P) receptor on lymphocytes, preventing their egress from peripheral lymph nodes (Figure 5.6). This redistribution of lymphocytes reduces the influx of pathogenic inflammatory cells into the CNS. Fingolimod also binds S1P receptors on neural cells within the CNS, although little is known about the downstream effects of this interaction.

TABLE 5.3

New generation disease-modifying therapy

Drug	Dose/ administration	Frequency	Side effects	Comments
Natalizumab (Tysabri)	300 mg i.v.	Monthly	Infusion reactions (< 2%) Hepatic dysfunction (< 0.5%) PML (< 0.5%, risk stratified) Neutralizing antibodies	PML risk sub-stratified with JC virus antibody testing (see Figure 5.5)
Fingolimod (Gilenya)	0.5 mg p.o.	Once daily	Cardiac: transient bradyarrhythmias requiring first-dose monitoring Ocular: 0.1% risk of retinal edema in first 3 months of therapy (requires ophthalmic review +/- OCT)	First oral disease-modifying therapy for MS
Teriflunomide (Aubagio)	7 mg p.o.	Once daily	Headaches, hepatic dysfunction and alopecia	Approved in the UK, USA and Australia*
Dimethyl fumarate (Tecfidera)	240 mg p.o.	Twice daily	Flushing (40%), diarrhea, headaches	Approved in Europe, the USA and Australia;* long-term safety data needed

*Approval pending in other countries at the time of publication.
i.v., intravenous; OCT, ocular coherence tomography; PML, progressive multifocal leukoencephalopathy; p.o., per os (by mouth).

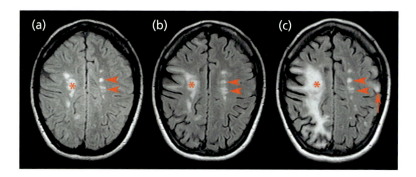

Figure 5.4 A 34-year-old female with relapsing remitting MS and subacute progressive left hemiparesis. She was treated with natalizumab for 2.8 years and had previous exposure to mitoxantrone for highly active MS. Axial fluid-attenuated inversion recovery (FLAIR) imaging shows evolving, diffuse signal change (asterisks) in the right hemisphere (a) 3 months before current presentation; (b) at baseline; and (c) at 6 months. Stable MS lesions are present in the left centrum semiovale (arrowheads). Early subcortical signal change related to progressive multifocal leukoencephalopathy (PML) is evident in the left hemisphere on the 6-month MRI scan (arrow). The diagnosis of PML was confirmed by the identification of JC virus (by polymerase chain reaction) in the cerebrospinal fluid at the time of the baseline MRI.

Fingolimod reduces the annualized relapse rate by 54% versus placebo at 2 years and by 52% versus intramuscular interferon beta-1a at 1 year. A modest relative reduction in the risk of disability progression confirmed after 3 and 6 months has also been demonstrated. Fingolimod also significantly reduced the rate of brain atrophy versus placebo at 2 years and versus intramuscular interferon beta-1a at 1 year. Extension studies confirm benefits on both disability and brain atrophy at 4 years' follow up.

However, there are rare and potentially serious side effects, including cardiac rhythm disturbances following the first dose, macular edema within the first 3 months of treatment, liver transaminase elevation and an increased risk of herpes simplex and varicella zoster viruses. Recommended safety measures include first-dose cardiac monitoring, ophthalmic surveillance, and vaccination

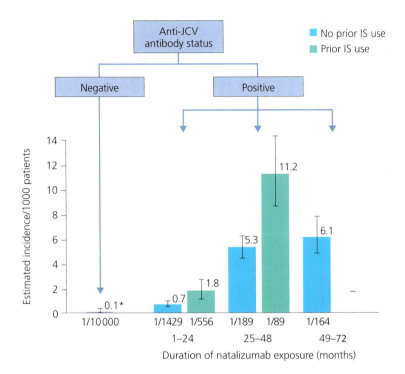

Figure 5.5 Risk stratification tool for progressive multifocal leukoencephalopathy (PML) based on anti-JC virus antibody status, prior immunosuppressant (IS) use and duration of natalizumab exposure. Data are from 343 confirmed cases of PML as of March 5, 2013. The highest risk, > 1/100, is in anti-JC virus antibody seropositive individuals previously exposed to immunosuppressive therapy and currently treated with natalizumab for more than 24 months. *The estimate of PML incidence in anti-JCV antibody negative patients is based on the assumption that all patients received at least 1 dose of natalizumab. – insufficient data. Adapted from data on file at Biogen Idec.

for varicella zoster virus before commencing treatment in seronegative patients. Although the long-term safety of fingolimod needs to be further established, the convenience of oral therapy and excellent patient tolerability should be included in the risk-benefit equation discussed with patients when deciding on an appropriate DMT.

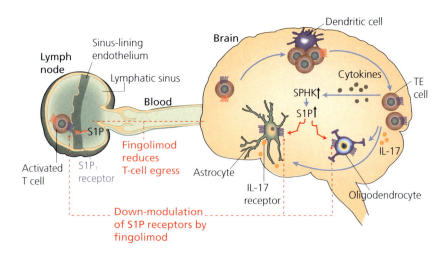

Figure 5.6 In the lymph nodes, activated T cells migrate into lymphatic sinuses in response to the sphingosine 1-phosphate (S1P) concentration gradient. S1P also modulates the permeability of the sinus-lining endothelium. Once in the CNS, differentiated effector T (TE) cells activate astrocytes through interleukin (IL)-17, directly kill neural cells and secrete inflammatory cytokines that activate sphingosine kinases (SPHKs). SPHKs increase the production of S1P, which may signal S1P receptors on many cell types to enhance neuroinflammation and gliosis. Fingolimod, which is structurally similar to S1P, initially binds to $S1P_1$ receptors, inhibiting egress from the lymph node; it also activates $S1P_1$ receptors on sinus-lining endothelial cells, enhancing the barrier function and reducing the transmigration of T cells into lymphatic sinuses. Fingolimod also acts as a highly potent antagonist, leading to internalization of $S1P_1$ receptors. As a result, the lymphocytes remain sequestered in the lymph node and do not invade the CNS. Furthermore, in the CNS, down-modulation of S1P receptors on neural cells may reduce hyperactivation, particularly of astrocytes, by excess S1P.

Teriflunomide. This once-daily oral therapy is licensed for use in relapsing forms of MS in the UK, USA and Australia. A hepatic metabolite of leflunomide, and an established therapy for rheumatoid arthritis, teriflunomide selectively and reversibly inhibits the mitochondrial enzyme dihydroorotate dehydrogenase (DHODH),

Clinical case: a 32-year-old woman (a single mother, working full time, with three children under the age of 8 years) with a 12-year history of MS, but relapse free for 6 years on interferon beta therapy, had a spinal relapse with bladder involvement. The patient's EDSS increased from 2.5 to 6.0 at the height of the relapse, but recovered to 4.0 following a brief course of intravenous methylprednisolone. Brain MRI demonstrated two enhancing lesions. She had also become increasingly distressed by persistent interferon beta-related injection-site reactions and flu-like symptoms.

Discussion: the patient experienced a significant spinal relapse despite conventional DMT, and MRI scans confirmed the presence of active cerebral disease. She was becoming less tolerant of interferon-beta injections, with the possible risk of decreased adherence to treatment. The patient's immunotherapy should be escalated, and natalizumab and fingolimod, both proven in Phase III clinical trials to have superior efficacy when compared to interferon beta, considered. While dimethyl fumarate also appears to have superior efficacy to conventional DMTs, the Phase III CONFIRM study, which included glatiramer acetate as a reference arm, was not designed to demonstrate superiority of dimethyl fumarate.

Given her complex social situation, it is likely that the 'distraction' and logistics of regular natalizumab infusions would detract from her quality of life; instead, a self-administered daily oral therapy would be advantageous. In this case, following a discussion of the potential risks, side effects and benefits, the patient elected to commence fingolimod.

which is required for de novo pyrimidine synthesis in proliferating lymphocytes. Slowly dividing or resting cells that rely on the salvage pathway for pyrimidine synthesis are relatively unaffected, largely preserving immune surveillance (Figure 5.7).

In Phase III clinical trials, teriflunomide, 14 mg daily, reduced the annualized MS relapse rate by 31.5–36.3% versus placebo, and reduced the risk of sustained (more than 12 weeks) disability

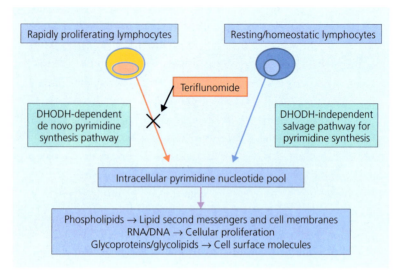

Figure 5.7 Teriflunomide inhibits de novo pyrimidine synthesis in proliferating lymphocytes by high affinity binding and inhibition of the mitochondrial enzyme dihydroorotate dehydrogenase (DHODH). Inhibition of pyrimidines leads to reduced T-cell proliferation, inhibition of DNA and RNA synthesis, reduced immunoglobulin secretion and inhibition of cytokines. Slowly dividing or resting cells that rely on the salvage pathway for pyrimidine synthesis are relatively unaffected.

progression by approximately 25–30%. Teriflunomide also had positive effects on MRI outcomes, although it has not been shown to slow the rate of brain atrophy versus placebo over 2 years.

Common side effects include nausea, diarrhea within the first few months of treatment, hair thinning and predominantly asymptomatic and transient elevation of alanine aminotransferase levels (monthly LFTs are required for the first 6 months of treatment). Rarely, treatment may be complicated by peripheral nerve toxicity requiring drug discontinuation. Teriflunomide is a potential teratogen and is contraindicated in pregnancy and in women of child-bearing potential not using reliable contraception. The drug has a long half-life (approximately 19 days), and in the case of inadvertent pregnancy (or plans to fall pregnant) on therapy, the drug must be rapidly 'washed out' with cholestyramine or activated charcoal.

Teriflunomide expands the treatment options available to patients with MS. As an oral therapy it may be an attractive first-line option for patients with mild to moderate disease, patients who are unable to tolerate interferon beta or glatiramer acetate, and specific patient groups such as those with cardiac comorbidities or diabetes mellitus in whom fingolimod may be contraindicated.

Dimethyl fumarate (BG-12). Approved in the USA, Canada, Australia and the EU, dimethyl fumarate, 240 mg twice daily, is an effective oral therapy that has shown promise as both a first-line treatment and escalation treatment for MS. Although the precise mode of action is unknown, dimethyl fumarate, following conversion to monomethyl fumarate, activates the nuclear factor (erythroid-derived 2)-like 2 (Nrf2) pathway, a cellular defense against oxidative stress (Figure 5.8).

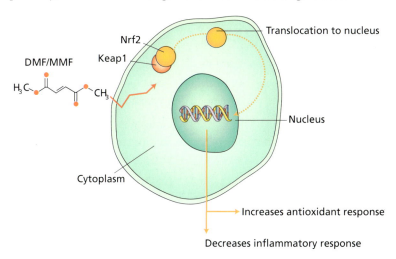

Figure 5.8 Under normal conditions, nuclear factor (erythroid-derived 2)-like 2 (Nrf2) is sequestered in the cytoplasm via kelch-like ECH-associated protein (Keap) 1. Dimethyl fumarate (DMF), following conversion to monomethyl fumarate (MMF), causes Nrf2 to translocate to the nucleus (imitating the physiological stress response), where it activates intrinsic antioxidant defense mechanisms and reduces the inflammatory response. Adapted from van Horssen J et al. *Biochem Biophys Acta* 2011;1812:141–150; Linker RA et al. *Brain* 2011;134:679–692; Scannevin R et al. *J Pharmacol Exp Ther* 2012;341:274–284.

Dimethyl fumarate may also have a direct Nrf2-independent anti-inflammatory effect.

In two Phase III trials (DEFINE and CONFIRM), dimethyl fumarate demonstrated a consistent reduction in annualized relapse rate of approximately 50% in patients with relapsing MS. Pooled data from these studies also showed a significant reduction in sustained disability progression at 2 years, and a 90% reduction in new gadolinium-enhancing lesions on MRI. Although glatiramer acetate was included as a reference arm in CONFIRM, and dimethyl fumarate appeared to produce better outcomes across all endpoints, the study was not powered to prove superiority.

No serious infections or malignancy have been noted, but long-term data in MS patients are lacking. The related compound 'Fumaderm' has been approved for the treatment of psoriasis for almost two decades in Germany. The most common side effect, flushing, occurs in approximately 40% of patients, but often settles in the first month of treatment and may be mitigated by taking dimethyl fumarate with food. Acetylsalicylic acid (ASA; aspirin), used before treatment with dimethyl fumarate, also diminishes flushing in patients with persistent symptoms. Gastrointestinal side effects are usually self-limiting and respond to antidiarrheal medicines such as loperamide. Dimethyl fumarate reduces the lymphocyte count by approximately 30%, and, rarely, may result in more profound lymphopenia. However, the need to establish long-term safety has been emphasized by recent reports of a possible association of treatment with fumaric acid esters and PML in the context of significant lymphopenia.

Immunosuppressive therapy

Traditional (cytotoxic) immunosuppressants are now rarely used in the treatment of MS, although they remain an option for those patients with relapsing MS whose condition is not adequately controlled by DMTs (see above). The imminent availability of more efficacious DMTs (e.g. alemtuzumab – see Chapter 6) will further expand the therapeutic arena for relapsing MS patients, and the future use of traditional immunosuppressants is likely to be restricted to rescue therapy in refractory cases.

Cyclophosphamide is used in patients with highly active relapsing remitting MS when DMTs are not effective in controlling the disease, and rarely in patients with progressive disease and evidence of ongoing 'inflammation', based either on the presence of superimposed relapses or MRI activity (gadolinium enhancement or increasing T2 lesion load). At a dose of 800–1000 mg administered monthly intravenously, cyclophosphamide is the mainstay of medical rescue treatment for refractory disease when all available DMTs have been exhausted.

The principal side effects of cyclophosphamide include bone marrow toxicity, hair loss and nausea/vomiting. Longer-term side effects include risk of secondary hematologic malignancy (leukemia/lymphoma).

Azathioprine. Mild immunosuppression with oral azathioprine, 2 mg/kg/day, was used in the 1990s in patients with frequent relapses requiring steroid treatment. Small early trials detected a 30% reduction in the annualized relapse rate. Some clinicians continue to use this therapy where discrete relapses cannot be observed but where steroid responsiveness is nonetheless demonstrated. However, there is a lack of level 1 evidence to support this approach, and the use of immunosuppressants may adversely affect the risk profile of subsequently prescribed new generation therapies such as natalizumab (see Figure 5.5, page 87).

Mitoxantrone, at a cumulative lifetime dose of less than 140 mg, effectively reduces relapses and has shown modest efficacy in reducing progressive disability in patients with secondary progressive MS. However, the efficacy of this treatment in patients with long-standing secondary progressive MS without superimposed relapses is questionable, and bone marrow toxicity, dose-dependent cardiotoxicity and an established 0.1–0.2% lifetime risk of acute myeloid leukemia significantly limits its clinical utility. Mitoxantrone has largely been supplanted by natalizumab in patients with highly active relapsing MS despite conventional DMT.

Treatment escalation strategy

Until the mid-2000s, the therapy of relapsing MS was limited to modestly effective conventional injectable DMT and, in refractory cases, cytotoxic agents. Over the past decade, the MS community has witnessed a remarkable transformation in the treatment landscape, with the introduction of novel efficacious oral and intravenous agents. While newer therapies such as fingolimod and natalizumab offer significant efficacy advantages over conventional DMT, their benefit must be weighed against a modest risk of complication. At present, quantifying the risks of therapy is confounded by the lack of long-term (10+ years) safety data for newer agents in MS cohorts.

For patients with mild to moderate disease, a treatment escalation strategy has been advocated, commencing with well-tolerated conventional DMT. Suboptimal clinical or radiological response to treatment should trigger consideration of second- and third-line treatments with greater expected efficacy. The simplified paradigm shown in Figure 5.9 represents the authors' views on how treatment might be escalated. In mild MS, most neurologists commence therapy with a relatively safe DMT such as interferon beta or glatiramer acetate, and escalate therapy to more efficacious treatment in patients who continue to exhibit significant clinical or MRI disease activity. The addition of the oral therapies to the MS treatment armamentarium has expanded the choice of DMT, particularly for patients with moderate disease, in countries where these medications are available. An increasing role for these treatments in mild disease is likely, but will depend on the availability of positive medium- and longer-term safety data. In patients with severe, or 'highly active' MS, natalizumab may be an appropriate choice, particularly when conventional therapies have failed, but also as first-line treatment in countries where this indication is available. While the place of alemtuzumab is yet to be clearly defined, it is likely to be used in patients with severe relapsing disease, especially those who continue to exhibit significant disease activity despite natalizumab or those with 'triple risk' for progressive multifocal leukoencephalopathy (see Figure 5.5). Patients who have failed other therapeutic avenues may, in selected

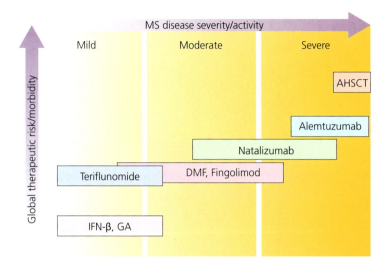

Figure 5.9 Authors' treatment escalation paradigm for relapsing remitting MS in relation to disease severity and activity, both clinical and radiological, balanced against the risks and side effects of therapy (see text). This does not take into account factors such as the patient's non-MS medical history, tolerance issues and personal preference. AHSCT, autologous hematopoietic stem cell transplantation; DMF, dimethyl fumarate; GA, glatiramer acetate; IFN-β, interferon beta.

cases and preferably within the context of a clinical trial, warrant high-dose immunosuppression (high-dose cyclophosphamide) without or with autologous hematopoietic stem cell transplantation, an experimental therapy with a mortality rate of 1–2% and significant associated morbidity.

The treatment escalation paradigm is clearly not applicable in all patients with relapsing MS, in particular those presenting with rapidly evolving disease. Considerations other than efficacy and safety, for instance a strong patient preference for oral therapy, may also dictate treatment choice in relapsing MS.

Key points – disease-modifying treatment

- Disease-modifying therapies ameliorate CNS inflammation in relapsing multiple sclerosis (MS), effectively reducing the relapse rate and the accumulation of new brain lesions identified on MRI.
- Early introduction of DMT, even at the stage of a clinically isolated syndrome, may be advantageous. Conversely, immune-directed DMT is not effective in patients with established secondary progressive MS.
- Newer DMTs, such as natalizumab and fingolimod, are significantly more effective than conventional injectable agents, but carry modest risks that must be considered when making treatment choices in individual patients.
- A treatment escalation strategy is appropriate for most patients with mild to moderate disease. Clinical and radiological parameters should be carefully monitored for evidence of disease activity in this paradigm.
- Early institution of efficacious newer generation therapies should be strongly considered in patients with rapidly evolving MS.
- Cytotoxic immunosuppression and hematopoietic stem cell transplantation are reserved for patients with MS that is refractory to available DMT.

Key references

Association of British Neurologists. Revised (2009) Association of British Neurologists' guidelines for prescribing in multiple sclerosis. www.theabn.org/abn/userfiles/file/ABN_MS_Guidelines_2009_Final(1).pdf

Cohen JA, Barkhof F, Comi G et al.; TRANSFORMS Study Group. Oral fingolimod or intramuscular interferon for relapsing multiple sclerosis. *N Engl J Med* 2010;362:402–15.

Gold R, Kappos L, Arnold DL et al.; DEFINE study investigators. Placebo-controlled phase 3 study of oral BG-12 for relapsing multiple sclerosis. *N Engl J Med* 2012;367: 1098–107.

Kappos L, Radue E-W, O'Connor P et al.; FREEDOMS Study Group. A placebo-controlled trial of oral fingolimod in relapsing multiple sclerosis. *N Engl J Med* 2010;362: 387–40.

Killestein J, Rudick RA, Polman CH. Oral treatments in multiple sclerosis. *Lancet Neurol* 2011;10:1026–34.

Kinkel RP, Dontchev M, Kollman C et al. Association between immediate initiation of intramuscular interferon beta-1a at the time of a clinically isolated syndrome and long-term outcomes: a 10-year follow-up of the Controlled High-Risk Avonex Multiple Sclerosis Prevention Study in Ongoing Neurological Surveillance Investigators. *Arch Neurol* 2012;69:183–90.

O'Connor P, Wolinsky JS, Confavreux C et al.; TEMSO Trial Group. Randomized trial of oral teriflunomide for relapsing multiple sclerosis. *N Engl J Med* 2011; 365:1293–303.

Polman CH, O'Connor PW, Havrdova E et al. A randomized, placebo-controlled trial of natalizumab for relapsing multiple sclerosis. *N Engl J Med* 2006;354:899–910.

Scalfari A, Nicholas R, Malik O, Muraro PA. Escalating immunotherapies for highly active multiple sclerosis: reviewing the evidence. *Current Medical Literature – Multiple Sclerosis*. 2010;2:61–73.

Dramatic advances in molecular and cellular biology over the last two decades have yielded numerous potential therapeutic targets in MS. Most therapeutic molecules that have entered clinical development interact with the adaptive immune system at one or more levels and therefore impact primarily upon the early relapsing phase of MS. Immune-directed therapies have little or no impact in the later progressive phase of the disease, which remains a major unmet treatment need. In the last 5–10 years, the emphasis of drug-discovery research in MS has begun to shift toward neuroprotection and the promotion of intrinsic central nervous system (CNS) repair mechanisms, with one such molecule, anti-Lingo 1 antibodies, entering a multinational Phase II trial program in 2013.

The proliferation of MS clinical trials has integrated scientists and neurologists within the new discipline of translational medicine, and fostered a critical and reciprocal exchange of expertise between these groups.

As the scope of this book does not allow a discussion on all aspects of these emerging therapies, we have restricted ourselves to treatments that are on the horizon, many of which have passed their Phase III clinical trial stage and are awaiting regulatory approval for licensing from the US Food and Drug Administration (FDA) or European Medicines Agency (EMA).

Monoclonal antibodies

Anti-CD52. Alemtuzumab, a monoclonal antibody directed against the cell surface molecule CD52, depletes the circulating lymphocytes (T and B cells) that effect inflammatory demyelination in MS. Alemtuzumab, 12 mg, is administered intravenously for 5 consecutive days, followed by a shorter course (3 consecutive days) in the second year of treatment with no interval therapy. Lymphocyte counts are restored months to years after treatment; in most cases, CD4+ T cells recover to approximately 200/mL by 6–9 months.

In three randomized trials, one Phase II trial (CAMMS223) and two Phase III trials (CARE-MS1, CARE-MS2), alemtuzumab significantly reduced relapse rate compared with the comparator subcutaneous interferon beta-1a (49–74% over 2–3 years). In the CAMMS223 and CARE-MS2 studies, alemtuzumab also showed a significantly greater benefit in terms of sustained disability progression versus the comparator (71% and 42%, respectively). However, alemtuzumab does not appear to reduce gradual deterioration in patients with secondary progressive disease. Many patients do not require further treatment (beyond the second course), with follow-up data on a subset of patients from the CAMMS223 study indicating benefit over interferon beta persisting for at least 5 years.

Alemtuzumab is most appropriate for patients with highly active disease or those with disease activity despite treatment with other disease-modifying therapies. A role for alemtuzumab in natalizumab-treated patients at high risk of progressive multifocal leukoencephalopathy (PML) (see Chapter 5) has yet to be defined.

Infusion requires hospital supervision, but can be performed in experienced outpatient infusion units in some patients. Infusion reactions are common but are ameliorated by concomitant administration of steroids and antihistamines. Autoimmunity, particularly the development of thyroid dysfunction (20%), is a commonly observed side effect of alemtuzumab therapy, and peaks 2–3 years after treatment. The risk of immune thrombocytopenic purpura is much lower (1–2%), but the condition may be fatal and requires monthly complete blood counts for at least 5 years after alemtuzumab treatment to facilitate prompt therapy with corticosteroids. Nephropathies, including anti-GBM antibody disease, are also a rare complication (0.3%). Early herpes virus infections are managed with prophylactic antiviral therapy and no serious opportunistic infections have been observed in clinical studies of patients with MS.

Anti-CD20. Monoclonal antibody therapies that target the CD20 cell surface molecule include rituximab, ocrelizumab and ofatumumab. These treatments induce prolonged depletion of B-cell precursors, while sparing mature plasma cells. Their mechanism of action in MS is unknown, but they may have an effect on B-cell trafficking into the CNS and, indirectly, on T-cell responses.

Rituximab and ocrelizumab have both dramatically suppressed MRI activity in Phase II studies compared with placebo, and a Phase III trial of ocrelizumab is ongoing. Notably, rituximab is often used off-label for the treatment of neuromyelitis optica, an inflammatory demyelinating disease of the CNS with a convincing humoral (antibody-mediated) pathogenesis.

Although no safety concerns have emerged in MS trial populations to date, ocrelizumab trials in rheumatoid arthritis and systemic lupus erythematosus have been discontinued because of an excess of opportunistic infections.

Anti-CD25. Daclizumab, a humanized monoclonal antibody, which binds to the cell surface molecule CD25, impairs the proliferation of autoreactive T cells, while expanding some natural killer cell populations. Daclizumab reduces the risk and severity of rejection in human organ transplantation. The mechanism of action in MS is unknown, but a regulatory effect on the immune system, mediated by natural killer cells, has been postulated.

In a Phase IIb trial (CHOICE), subcutaneously administered daclizumab reduced the number of gadolinium-enhancing lesions by 72% versus placebo at the higher of two doses. A larger Phase III trial (DECIDE) is under way.

Safety data from both the MS clinical trial program and the transplant literature are promising; transient thrombocytopenia, rash, lymphadenopathy and liver dysfunction have been reported.

Laquinimod

Laquinimod, a novel synthetic derivative of quinoline-3-carboxamide, is given once daily as oral therapy. Following successful preclinical studies in animal models of neuroinflammation, it has been studied in two Phase III trials, where it exerted a modest (23%) non-significant reduction in annualized relapse rate but a significant improvement in the progression of disability and whole brain volume loss versus placebo.

Other than a transient elevation of liver enzymes, laquinimod has exhibited no concerning side effects in the clinical trial program to date. The apparent disjunct between an effect on relapses and disability progression/brain volume loss suggests that laquinimod may have a unique mechanism of action, possibly mediated through a direct effect on innate immune cells in the CNS. Additional Phase III trials are under way to establish the efficacy of laquinimod and define a potential place for this agent in MS treatment.

Stem cell therapy

The application of stem cell therapies to MS is perhaps more frequently raised by patients with the condition than their neurologists. However, both conventional (hematopoietic) and novel stem cell approaches (Table 6.1) offer potential new therapeutic avenues for MS, especially in patients whose disease is refractory to current disease-modifying treatments.

Autologous hemopoietic stem cell transplantation (AHSCT) is in effect a means of 'rebooting' the immune system by ablating bone marrow and repopulating it with the patient's own hemopoietic (bone marrow) stem cells. While there are no Phase III randomized controlled trials of AHSCT, early studies in MS indicate a greater than 90% reduction in

TABLE 6.1

Potential stem cell therapies in multiple sclerosis

Stem cell	Immune regeneration	(Neural) tissue regeneration
Embryonic	✓	✓
Embryonic/fetal neural precursor cells	?	✓
Adult neural	?	✓
Bone marrow-derived		
Hematopoietic	✓	?
Mesenchymal	✓ (modulation)	?

relapse rate compared with pretreatment levels of disease activity. Dramatic MRI responses to AHSCT have also been reported. Impressive clinical and radiological efficacy in patients with severe active disease comes at the cost of significant morbidity/mortality, associated in large part with the intensity of the chemotherapeutic conditioning regimen (2–4% in specialized units). At present, the technique is usually reserved for patients with aggressive disease who have failed to respond to other treatments. There is no evidence that immunoablative therapy will be efficacious in gradually progressive forms of MS. International multicenter clinical trials are starting, which should help to define a population of patients in whom the risk/benefit analysis weighs in favor of this treatment approach.

Mesenchymal stem cell transplantation. The concept of self-renewing multipotent stem cells (i.e. cells that can differentiate into any cell type) as the basis for tissue repair in the nervous system, which has a physiologically limited regenerative capacity in adults, is extremely attractive. Mesenchymal tissue can be harvested from bone marrow, placental or adipose tissue, and multipotent mesenchymal stem cells expanded and purified in vitro. From only a few stem cells, billions/trillions of self-regenerating stem cells can be grown using specific nutrients (growth factors) and then readministered to the patient (intravenously or intrathecally) without the need for toxic conditioning regimens. Evidence from preclinical studies in experimental autoimmune encephalomyelitis (EAE) models supports both an immunomodulatory and neuroprotective role for mesenchymal stem cells.

Experimental (Phase I/II) studies have demonstrated the feasibility of this approach in humans, with no serious adverse reactions reported to date. Although there have been only a few dozen patients in open-label studies so far, early data suggest that these cells may have an ameliorating effect on inflammation in MS patients. The capacity of these cells to differentiate into physiologically functional neural tissue (remyelination/regeneration) is yet to be determined.

Vitamin D

Low vitamin D levels are epidemiologically associated with an increased risk of developing MS (see Chapter 1). Several small studies have examined the potential of dietary vitamin D supplementation, 1000–4000 IU/day, to ameliorate relapse frequency in MS and yielded inconsistent results. Larger studies, in particular the placebo-controlled PrevANZ study of vitamin D supplementation in patients with a clinically isolated syndrome, are awaited with interest. In the interim, many patients with MS and low or low–normal vitamin D levels are empirically treated with dietary vitamin D supplementation. Studies of vitamin D supplementation in individuals predisposed to MS (e.g. those with a family history of MS) are also forthcoming.

Anti-lingo antibody

Promoting repair in MS is, so far, an unexplored sphere of MS therapy. Lingo antagonists promote oligodendrocyte differentiation and myelination in vitro and in animal models of demyelination. The first multinational Phase II trial of anti-lingo 1 antibodies in patients with acute optic neuritis commenced in 2013. Ultimately, therapies that successfully promote remyelination and repair may be applicable across the spectrum of MS subtypes, including progressive forms of the disease.

Key points – emerging therapies

- A greater understanding of MS pathogenesis, from genetic susceptibilities and mechanisms of immune-mediated tissue injury through to the molecular basis of impaired tissue repair, has facilitated the development of new treatments for the disease.
- The spectrum of disease-modifying therapies available to the MS clinician is expected to significantly expand over the next 5–10 years.
- Therapies currently under study include novel small-molecule immunomodulators, targeted immune-directed monoclonal antibodies, hematopoietic and mesenchymal stem-cell therapies, vitamin D supplementation and molecules that promote remyelination and repair.
- Treatments such as alemtuzumab, B-cell directed monoclonal antibody treatments and autologous hematopoietic stem cell transplant may be appropriate for the treatment of patients with highly active relapsing disease that has not responded to other disease-modifying therapies.
- Laquinimod may have a novel mechanism of action that targets innate immune cells; it appears to impact disability progression and brain volume loss more than relapse rate.
- Anti-lingo antibody is the first remyelination-promoting therapy to reach Phase II clinical trials in MS. Treatments that overcome molecular obstacles to remyelination may complement immune-directed therapies for MS in the future.

Key references

Brown JWL, Coles AJ. Alemtuzumab: evidence for its potential in relapsing–remitting multiple sclerosis. *Drug Des Devel Ther* 2013;7:131–8.

CAMMS223 Trial Investigators, Coles AJ, Compston DA, Selmaj KW et al. Alemtuzumab vs. interferon beta-1a in early multiple sclerosis. *N Engl J Med* 2008;359:1786–801.

Comi G, Jeffery D, Kappos L et al. Placebo-controlled trial of oral laquinimod for multiple sclerosis. *N Engl J Med* 2012;366:1000–9.

Freedman MS. Present and emerging therapies for multiple sclerosis. *Continuum (Minneap Minn)* 2013;19(4 Multiple Sclerosis):968–91.

Gold R, Giovannoni G, Selmaj K et al. Daclizumab high-yield process in relapsing-remitting multiple sclerosis (SELECT): a randomised, double-blind, placebo-controlled trial. *Lancet* 2013;381:2167–75.

Hauser SL, Waubant E, Arnold DL et al. B-cell depletion with rituximab in relapsing-remitting multiple sclerosis. *N Engl J Med* 2008;358:676–88.

Holloman JP, Ho CC, Hukki A et al. The development of hematopoietic and mesenchymal stem cell transplantation as an effective treatment for multiple sclerosis. *Am J Stem Cells* 2013;2:95–107.

Kappos L, Li D, Calabresi PA et al. Ocrelizumab in relapsing-remitting multiple sclerosis: a phase 2, randomised, placebo-controlled, multicentre trial. *Lancet* 2011;378:1779–87.

Oh J, Calabresi PA. Emerging injectable therapies for multiple sclerosis. *Lancet Neurol* 2013;12:1115–26.

Rieckmann P, Traboulsee A, Devonshire V, Oger J. Escalating immunotherapy of multiple sclerosis. *Ther Adv Neurol Disord* 2008;1:181–92.

Saccardi R, Freedman MS, Sormani MP et al. A prospective, randomized, controlled trial of autologous haematopoietic stem cell transplantation for aggressive multiple sclerosis: a position paper. *Mult Scler* 2012;18:825–34.

Pregnancy

Multiple sclerosis (MS) often affects young women between the ages of 20 and 40 years at a time when they are most likely to be planning a family. It is important to ask patients with MS about their plans for pregnancy early so as to balance medical interventions against the risks to the baby and mother; this should, ideally, result in planned pregnancies. Both obstetric and neurological teams should be involved throughout the pregnancy, although the obstetric management is rarely affected directly by the neurological issues. In particular, the mode of delivery (natural versus interventional) is not generally an issue. Suggestions that general anesthetics or epidural cannulas can influence neurological status have not been borne out by the clinical evidence.

It is important to note that while a diagnosis of MS may influence pregnancy planning, it does not affect fertility. However, sexual function may be adversely affected by multiple factors including psychological perceptions regarding body image and physical factors including genitourinary dysfunction and altered sensation.

Pregnancy is a physiological state that involves relative immunologic modulation. Pregnancy appears to have a favorable effect on MS, with reduced rates of relapse, especially in the third trimester. This is usually accompanied by a compensatory rise in relapse rates in the postpartum period (the 3 months after delivery), so that overall pregnancy is largely neutral in terms of its effect on relapse rate. Previous reports of postpartum deterioration in MS have not been seen in robust studies, and pregnancy does not appear to affect disease progression.

Possible reasons why pregnancy affects relapse rate include:
- immunologic: balance of Th-1 (promotes inflammation)/Th-2 (ameliorates inflammation – see Chapter 2) response
- hormonal: estriol is an estrogen that is only found in pregnancy; it may have a beneficial effect in terms of reducing relapse rate
- elevated calcitriol (1,25-dihydroxyvitamin D3) levels occur during normal pregnancy.

Contraception. The progesterone-only or combined oral contraceptive pills have no known adverse effect on MS.

Treating relapses in pregnancy. There are no guidelines on the treatment of relapse in pregnancy. All treatment options should be discussed on a case-by-case basis. Although there is limited information on the effect of steroid therapy in pregnancy, steroids are generally considered to be relatively safe. The placenta is responsible for the metabolism of methylprednisolone, thus minimizing fetal exposure.

Disease-modifying treatments

Interferon beta. While there are limited data, pregnancy registers do not suggest a teratogenic effect of interferon beta in humans, but an increased rate of spontaneous abortion and low birth weight has been reported in small studies. Patients who become pregnant while taking interferon-beta therapy are advised to stop the treatment for at least the remainder of the first trimester as the effects on development of the fetal immune system are unknown. Pregnancy should be planned and the potential risks and benefits of therapy discussed in advance. In general, cessation of interferon-beta prior to conception is recommended. In select patients with active relapsing MS, the authors may advise maintenance of interferon beta until pregnancy is confirmed.

Glatiramer acetate. Similarly, limited data suggest neither an increased risk of spontaneous abortion nor a teratogenic effect of glatiramer acetate. In patients with active relapsing MS, maintenance of glatiramer acetate through pregnancy has been advocated by some groups; the risk-benefit analysis should be assessed and discussed with the individual patient.

Natalizumab. Prospective follow-up of the small number of patients with MS exposed to the drug during pregnancy has not revealed any significant increase in teratogenicity and the propensity to relapse after cessation of natalizumab increases substantially beyond 3 months. The authors therefore recommend maintenance of natalizumab until pregnancy is confirmed in select patients.

Other disease-modifying therapies. There are limited data regarding fingolimod and dimethyl fumarate in pregnancy; however, recommendations mandate cessation of treatment prior to conception.

Teriflunomide is a potential teratogen and must not be used in pregnancy or by women of childbearing potential who are not using reliable contraception. The drug has a long half-life and in the case of inadvertent pregnancy (or plans to fall pregnant) on therapy, rapid 'wash out' with cholestyramine or activated charcoal is required.

Azathioprine is considered relatively safe in pregnancy, but methotrexate is associated with an increased risk of congenital malformations and spontaneous abortion, and should be avoided. These therapies were once widely adopted as MS treatments in Europe, but are now only rarely used following the introduction of natalizumab and fingolimod.

Breastfeeding. The ability to breastfeed is typically not affected in patients with MS and does not affect the risk of relapse in the postpartum period. The relative concentrations of disease-modifying therapies within breast milk are not known, but it is generally recommended not to use these drugs whilst breastfeeding. Short courses of corticosteroids are not contraindicated during breastfeeding. In patients with clinically or radiologically active disease in the postpartum period, consideration should be given to cessation of breastfeeding and re-institution of disease-modifying therapy.

Other comorbidities associated with pregnancy. As pregnancy is a prothrombotic state, appropriate thromboprophylaxis should be considered in patients with significant immobility.

Urinary tract infections are more common in pregnancy, and are likely to be more frequent and more severe where there is a pre-existing neurogenic bladder. This may require more regular intermittent self-catheterization and/or the use of prophylactic antibiotics.

A small proportion of patients with MS with pre-existing mobility difficulties or significant spasticity may experience worsening due to increased bodyweight.

In those with significant spinal cord involvement, autonomic dysfunction can rarely cause sympathomimetic overactivity leading to uncontrolled hypertension. Precipitating factors (e.g. vaginal examinations, catheter blockages) are best avoided. Occasionally, specific antihypertensives are required, and epidural anesthesia may need to be employed if labor is induced.

Key points – pregnancy

- Multiple sclerosis does not affect fertility.
- The oral contraceptive pill (OCP) does not affect MS, and MS does not affect the efficacy of the OCP.
- Ideally, pregnancy in patients with MS should be planned and managed with both obstetric and neurological input.
- Pregnancy may result in reduced relapse risk, especially in the third trimester, but does not affect the overall progression of MS.
- Relapses during pregnancy should be treated on a case-by-case basis with specialist input.
- Although data are limited, there is no evidence of teratogenicity with interferon beta, glatiramer acetate or natalizumab therapy.
- In general, interferon-beta and glatiramer acetate therapy should be stopped when pregnancy is confirmed. In patients with highly active MS, an argument can be made to maintain glatiramer acetate provided the patient is cognizant of the potential risks.
- Methotrexate and teriflunomide must not be used in pregnancy. Teriflunomide has a long half-life and must be appropriately 'washed out' before conception.
- There are insufficient data regarding fingolimod and dimethyl fumarate; however, cessation of these therapies prior to conception is recommended.
- Thromboprophylaxis should be considered in patients with MS who have significant immobility.
- The ability to breastfeed is not affected unless the patient has significant motor impairment. Disease-modifying therapies should in general not be used when breastfeeding.

Children

Pediatric MS is defined as MS with onset below the age of 16–18 years (depending on the study). This group makes up approximately 3–4% of all people with MS. The majority of children with MS (> 95%) have the relapsing remitting subtype of the disease. Secondary progression is very unusual in the pediatric population and rarely occurs within 15 years of diagnosis.

Epidemiology. MS is more common in girls than boys diagnosed over the age of 6. Below this age, there are proportionally more boys than girls with the disease.

Initial presentation. Most children have a multifocal presentation, with more than one anatomic site affected. Monofocal presentations are more common in adolescents. Presenting symptoms are shown in Table 7.1.

Differential diagnosis. A presentation of multifocal disease can be difficult to differentiate from acute disseminated encephalomyelitis (ADEM). ADEM is a monophasic inflammatory condition that usually presents with headache, encephalopathy, fever and meningism. It has a polysymptomatic presentation that often follows antecedent infection or vaccination. Clinical features and/or neuroimaging confirm the presence of multiple (inflammatory) CNS lesions of the same or a

TABLE 7.1

Presenting symptoms of multiple sclerosis in children

Motor dysfunction	27–30%
Cerebellar symptoms	11–28%
Sensory symptoms	15–27%
Brainstem syndromes	19–22%
Optic neuritis (more common in Asia)	10–22%
Transverse myelitis	< 10%

similar age. Slow or incomplete recovery is not uncommon, with residual deficits such as epilepsy, learning difficulties and behavioral disturbances. ADEM can only be confidently distinguished from MS by adequate follow up. In this regard, it is important to recognize there is often a long period between the first and second episode of MS in children who are under 10 years old at the time of symptom onset. Other differential diagnoses in children are shown in Table 7.2.

Risk in children. The risk of clinically definite MS (as demonstrated by a second clinical episode) after a childhood clinically isolated syndrome approaches 50% within 3 years if focal neurological features are present at onset. The risk is almost 30% in children with an encephalopathic ADEM-like presentation (Table 7.3).

Clinically isolated optic neuritis carries a lower risk of MS – about 13% by 10 years and 22% by 23 years. In children of Asian origin with clinically isolated optic neuritis, particular consideration should be given to alternative diagnoses such as neuromyelitis optica (NMO), for which specific immunotherapy may be indicated.

TABLE 7.2

Differential diagnosis of multiple sclerosis in children

- Acute disseminated encephalomyelitis
- CNS infection
- Neuromyelitis optica*
- Other CNS inflammatory disorders (vasculitis, sarcoidosis, histiocytoses)
- Metabolic disorders (inborn errors of metabolism and mitochondrial disorders)
- Dysmyelination syndromes including adrenoleukodystrophy, metachromatic leukodystrophy and Pelizaeus–Merzbacher disease
- Neoplasia (especially CNS lymphoma)

*In addition to optic nerve and spinal cord involvement, there may be additional cerebral and brainstem involvement leading to encephalopathy, seizures and intractable vomiting and hiccups.
CNS, central nervous system.

TABLE 7.3

Factors that predict a subsequent diagnosis of MS after childhood CIS

- Over 10 years old at onset
- No cognitive change at onset
- Family history of optic neuritis or MS
- Abnormal MRI scan (as in adults)

CIS, clinically isolated syndrome.

Diagnostic tests

Magnetic resonance imaging. As in adults, the morphology and distribution of inflammatory brain lesions, particularly those oriented perpendicular to the long axis of the corpus callosum, may help to predict or diagnose MS in children. The presence of both enhancing and non-enhancing lesions at presentation increases the likelihood of dissemination of lesions in time. However, MRI does not reliably distinguish MS from ADEM, and the sensitivity of MRI in children under the age of 10 years is relatively low. MRI does help to exclude differential diagnoses and should be performed in all children in whom an inflammatory CNS event is suspected.

Cerebral spinal fluid. Lumbar puncture is performed in many children, primarily to rule out an infective meningo-encephalitis. Although a mild CSF pleocytosis is common, the total white cell count is rarely more than 30 leukocytes/mm³. Oligoclonal bands (see page 41) are found in 90% of children with MS, although not all children are positive at the time of the initial lumbar puncture. They are less frequently found in children with ADEM or NMO.

Serology. There is no serological test for MS. The serum of children with NMO usually contains antibodies to the water channel aquaporin 4. MS may present following viral or other infection and positive serological tests do not distinguish MS from ADEM, which is more commonly preceded by infection ('post-infectious encephalomyelitis'). Serological tests for specific CNS infections may be relevant in some patients, especially in areas where Lyme disease (neuroborreliosis) is endemic.

Electrophysiology. Multimodal evoked potentials are useful to help to establish disease dissemination in space and time; however, these have been largely supplanted by MRI in the modern era.

Disabling symptoms and outcome. Fatigue contributing to absence from school is noted in 40% of children with MS, and seizures occur in approximately 5%. Cognitive impairment is found in approximately 30% of children with MS. Although there is relative sparing of verbal fluency, deficits in general cognition, visuomotor integration and memory have been noted.

Kurtzke's expanded disability status scale (EDSS) is the most common measure of disability in people with MS (see Table 3.9). The EDSS score in children rises with disease duration. On average, it takes children with MS 10 years longer to reach EDSS 7–10 than adults with MS. Progression to the secondary progressive stage of MS is primarily determined by disease duration.

Management principles. In children, it is important to ensure that the diagnosis of MS is firm before proceeding with treatment. A multidisciplinary approach is essential, and clear communication with children with MS and their parents is paramount. It is important that there is an understanding of the course of the disease, and that children are able to recognize the symptoms of relapse from an early age.

Psychologists, physiotherapists, occupational therapists, speech and language therapists and specialist teaching staff all have an important role in the management of children with MS. It is important to consider the social and educational difficulties that arise in the context of a diagnosis of MS during childhood and adolescence. The pediatric and adult neurology teams must work together, especially during the adolescent years when acceptance of the disease and adherence to treatment may prove difficult.

It is important to counsel adolescents with regards to pregnancy and contraception if they are sexually active.

Relapse therapy. Corticosteroid therapy is used for treatment of disabling relapses. Although there are no trial data to support the use of steroids in children, intravenous or oral methylprednisolone is used empirically up to a maximum of 1 g per dose for 3–5 days. Intravenous immunoglobulin (Ig) has been used, with case series stating benefit from doses of 2 g/kg administered over 2–5 days. Anecdotal reports suggest that, as in adults, plasma exchange can be useful in severe steroid-refractory relapses.

Disease-modifying therapies. Conventional disease-modifying therapies (interferon beta and glatiramer acetate) are reported, in small open-label studies, to confer a similar benefit on relapse rate to that observed in adults (see page 76). Similar side effects are also observed, although liver dysfunction related to the use of interferon beta may be more common in children. As in adults, glatiramer acetate can cause self-limited episodes of flushing and tachycardia in some children, and the patient and their family should be aware of this benign though often frightening side effect. Natalizumab has been reported to be highly effective in small case series of children with aggressive relapsing MS, although in some countries it is not licensed for use in individuals under 18 years of age. There are currently no data regarding the use of fingolimod, dimethyl fumarate or teriflunomide in children.

Key points – children

- MS is not common in children.
- Most children with MS have the relapsing remitting type.
- Children more often present with multiple symptoms.
- Differential diagnoses, including acute disseminated encephalomyelitis (ADEM), CNS infection and neuromyelitis optica (NMO), should be considered.
- The accumulation of disability is slower in children with MS than in adults.
- Multidisciplinary involvement is an important aspect of therapy, with special focus on the psychological aspects of chronic disease in childhood and adolescence.

Full blood count and liver function tests should be carried out monthly for the first 6 months of interferon-beta therapy, then every 3–6 months. Thyroid function should also be checked annually.

The elderly

Thanks to improvements in supportive and multidisciplinary care, patients with MS can expect to have a near-normal life expectancy. Elderly patients with MS may have either longstanding 'conventional' adult-onset MS, or the late-onset MS subtype, which is defined as MS with symptom onset after the age of 50 years. In the latter group, a disproportionately higher number of patients have the primary progressive type of MS. Late-onset MS commonly presents with motor symptoms, while optic neuritis and sensory symptoms are relatively uncommon. This group has a higher rate of depression, and suicidal ideation is not uncommon. In one study, the cause of death in 15% of elderly patients with MS was suicide.

Aging also widens the list of differential diagnoses, and the presence of comorbid illnesses in this group affects disability and medical options for treatment.

Treatment. Patients in this age group are rarely considered for clinical trials, so there is sparse evidence available, but the disease-modifying therapies offered to elderly persons with relapsing MS do not differ substantially from those offered to younger adults with the condition. It is important to monitor renal and hepatic function closely in older patients receiving drug therapies because of their potential for comorbid disease. This age group is also more vulnerable to the infective and potential neoplastic side effects of newer immunosuppressive therapies. Similarly, cardiac comorbidities may be relevant in elderly patients considering fingolimod therapy.

Screening for adequate treatment of depression is also important, and a thorough assessment of the patient's social support is necessary. In this regard, a multidisciplinary team is best placed to manage the elderly patient with MS. The role of physiotherapists and occupational therapists in falls prevention is especially important.

Key points – the elderly

- Late-onset MS is defined as MS with symptom onset after the age of 50 years.
- Primary progressive MS is more common in late-onset MS than in younger patients.
- Comorbid illness affects disability, treatment choice and treatment monitoring.
- Depression is common and should be screened for at each review.

Key references

Awadl A, Stuvel O. Multiple sclerosis in the elderly patient. *Drugs Aging* 2010;27:283–94.

Banwell B, Ghezzi A, Bar-Or A et al. Multiple sclerosis in children: clinical diagnosis, therapeutic strategies, and future directions. *Lancet Neurol* 2007;6:887–902.

Lee M, O'Brien P. Pregnancy and multiple sclerosis. *J Neurol Neurosurg Psychiatry* 2008;79:1308–11.

Vukusic S, Hutchinson M, Hours M et al., The Pregnancy In Multiple Sclerosis Group. Pregnancy and multiple sclerosis (the PRIMS study): clinical predictors of post-partum relapse. *Brain* 2004;127(Pt 6):1353–60.

Yeh EA, Chitnis T, Krupp L et al. Pediatric multiple sclerosis. *Nature Rev Neurol* 2009;5:621–31.

Lifestyle considerations and the multidisciplinary team

Counseling

Multiple sclerosis (MS) is a clinically heterogeneous condition, and the advice we give must be tailored to the individual patient's disease phenotype, medical history and social circumstance. Counseling should not only involve what we know about the disease itself but also what effect MS will have on all aspects of life, including career, family, travel, insurance and the concerns raised by having a new diagnosis of MS. Patients are keen to know whether their life expectancy will be affected and whether the disease is transmissible to their children (Table 8.1). The diagnosis may affect their employment status, whether they decide to have children and where they decide to live. There are often questions about whether they could have avoided the disease by changing their behavior in any way.

The multidisciplinary team

Neurologist. The medical team is important in coordinating multidisciplinary patient care. It is the neurologist's role to make a firm diagnosis as early as possible in the course of the disease. Once the diagnosis has been established, the neurologist must ensure that the patient is fully informed of all approved treatment options and understands both their benefits and risks. Neurologists are also well-positioned to provide patients with the opportunity to participate in local clinical trials of emerging disease-modifying and symptomatic therapies. Neurologists strive to understand more about the pathophysiology and evolution of MS, and translate this information to the clinical care of their patients.

General practitioner/family doctor. The primary care provider will be able to coordinate all the threads of care for a patient with MS throughout their life. They will have access to allied healthcare professionals, and will be able to refer to specialists (neurologist,

TABLE 8.1

Questions that patients often ask

Is the disease hereditary?

Genetic factors play a part in determining susceptibility to MS, but there is no single causative gene (see Table 1.1, page 11).

What is the effect of pregnancy?

Relapse risk may diminish in the latter stages of pregnancy, but does increase during the postpartum period (up to 3 months after birth). There are no data to suggest that MS has an adverse effect on the fetus, or that the long-term outcome of MS is influenced by the patient's obstetric history.

Can I have vaccinations?

Yes. There is no firm evidence that single vaccinations trigger an acute exacerbation of MS or alter its long-term outcome. Infection may itself be a trigger for MS relapse, and patients at risk of specific vaccine-preventable disease should, in general, be vaccinated. Patients treated with any form of immunosuppressive therapy should not receive live-attenuated vaccinations. The efficacy of vaccination may also be reduced in patients receiving immunotherapy.

Can I have an anesthetic?

Yes. There is no evidence that general, regional (including epidural) or local anesthesia trigger exacerbations of the disease.

Should I avoid dental procedures?

No. Dental procedures do not affect the course of the condition, and no special precautions are needed for most people with MS. In addition, there is no evidence to justify the removal of intact mercury-containing amalgam fillings to improve MS.

Should I go on a special diet?

There is little evidence to support any requirement for dietary change in patients with MS. Maintaining an ideal bodyweight with a balanced, low-fat diet and good conditioning is important.

CONTINUED

TABLE 8.1 (CONTINUED)

Should I have oxygen therapy?

No. Although an early study suggested that hyperbaric (high-pressure) oxygen therapy may be beneficial, the findings have not been supported by subsequent research. Known side effects include cataracts, seizures and pneumothorax.

Acceptance of the disease is further hampered by the lack of a curative therapy, and patients' reticence to commit to long-term therapies that may not be without risk leads many to explore alternative therapies before commencing prescribed disease-modifying treatments. Evidence of benefit for alternative therapies is lacking, and they are not discussed further. Treatment decisions need to be made at each stage of the disease, and as healthcare providers we must offer clear realistic advice.

urologist, obstetrician, psychiatrist, rehabilitation therapist) for the wide range of symptoms and concerns that patients may have at different stages of the disease. As care providers over a lifetime, they have a unique insight into the needs of the individual. Good communication within the healthcare support team will ensure a well-integrated approach to the management of MS and its resulting morbidity.

Specialist nurse. In large centers, the MS specialist nurse has become an integral and invaluable member of the multidisciplinary team. Trained MS nurses are a reliable source of information about all aspects of MS, and can provide patients with practical advice on living with the condition. The specialist nurse can counsel people who have recently received a diagnosis of MS, and they are usually easy to contact when questions arise outside the consultation. After diagnosis, specialist nurses are often the first port of call when a patient is concerned that they may be having a relapse. They can provide prompt clinical assessment and, where necessary, review.

The MS specialist nurse is well placed to explain the practical aspects associated with all disease-modifying therapies to patients considering immunotherapy. Traditionally, training in the use of injectable therapies has been a principal role for the MS nurse. In the modern therapeutic era, specialist MS nurses also supervise patients who receive infusions and coordinate and run first-dose clinics for fingolimod. They can be called upon if adverse effects occur, or if patients are having difficulty adhering to a particular therapy. Finally, specialist nurses help patients deal with the social impact of MS and can provide a link to other services such as social workers and clinical psychologists.

Physiotherapist. The physiotherapist is vital in helping patients to remain mobile for as long as possible, and plays a crucial synergistic role in the management of spasticity. As well as providing the patient with specific exercises that help prevent the development of contractures and pressure sores, the physiotherapist can offer practical advice and training in falls prevention. Physiotherapists are a valuable source of encouragement, and help to optimize the functional abilities of patients with MS, maintaining a range of movement and limb strength for as long as possible.

Speech and language therapist. The SALT team are highly skilled in the assessment of speech and swallowing. They can aid communication in patients who have severe dysarthria, and also delineate the nature of swallowing problems in MS. They can recommend dietary changes and actions to maximize swallowing and to minimize the risk of aspiration. They are able to identify when swallowing has deteriorated to high risk levels, and can recommend when institutional enteral feeding should be considered.

Occupational therapist. The occupational therapist works with the patient to allow them to remain independent for as long as possible. They will assess functional ability and evaluate how activities of daily living are carried out. They can then recommend training or equipment to make life easier, and to allow a person to return home or to a working environment.

Occupational therapists can install handrails in the home, and can plan conversion of bathrooms to 'wet' rooms to minimize the risk of falls. They will assess how safe it is for certain functions to be carried out (e.g. boiling a kettle) and either recommend equipment or behavioral changes (avoidance) to ensure the patient's safety.

Dietitian. The dietitian can help to plan a diet that is high in fiber to improve bowel function in patients with constipation. Dietitians also plan diets designed to maintain health, particularly in patients who require an exclusion diet for other reasons (e.g. gluten intolerance). In advanced MS associated with weight loss and swallowing difficulties, they may design a diet that is tailored to the needs of the individual. There may be a greater risk of osteoporosis in patients with MS, for which the dietitian can recommend a diet rich in calcium or, when required, supplements such as vitamin D and calcium. Dietitians also manage enteral feeding if a gastrostomy becomes necessary.

Social worker. It is important that people with MS receive financial, housing and other practical assistance when required. Patients may not always be aware of their entitlements, and for many reasons they may struggle with completing forms. Social workers have an understanding of the social system of their country and are able to advise and assist people with MS to ensure that they receive appropriate assistance from the government and relevant non-governmental organizations. Rehousing to incorporate the needs of the patient and their family requires vital input from social workers. They are also able to monitor for any signs of abuse of vulnerable people, and act to protect those in need of help.

Other valuable members of the team. Psychologists can assess the patient's mood and cognition, and assist with educational support. Continence nurses can assess bladder problems, assist with continence training, provide advice on pelvic floor exercises and urinary aids, and ensure appropriate maintenance of catheters to minimize infection.

Patient rights – education and employment

MS affects people mainly between the ages of 20 and 40 years, generally the most productive time of their lives, especially with regards to children and career. Some people are diagnosed early in their career, and it is important that they are not discriminated against on the basis of the diagnosis. In the early stages of the disease, disability may not be visible but symptoms such as fatigue and cognitive dysfunction can be disabling. People with MS may encounter a lack of understanding about the severity of the disability, and they may face the dilemma of when to disclose the condition to their employers. Consequently, concerns regarding employment can become a great source of stress.

Maintaining a place in education and the workforce has numerous financial, physical and psychological benefits. It is therefore important that people with MS receive appropriate information and support to assist them to stay in education and employment for as long as possible. It is important to highlight to patients that they are not obliged to disclose their illness to everyone at work, but as MS can affect physical, cognitive and emotional functioning they are likely to need support in the workplace as the disease progresses. The specific diagnosis does not need to be disclosed to employers at interview (although disability will usually need to be). In the UK, for example, employers must be informed of the diagnosis if the employment is in the armed forces, on a plane or on a ship. Some employment contracts specifically request disclosure of diagnoses like MS, as most employers need to know about specific disabilities in order to adhere to the relevant laws in their country.

Employers have an obligation to aid employees as much as possible to remain in employment. Even if there is little disability at the time of employment, employers will need to allow time off to recover from relapses or to attend hospital appointments. If 'reasonable adjustments' can be made to the workplace setting to enable the employee to continue working, in many countries the employer is required by law to make these. The nature of these adjustments will depend on the individual circumstances and what is considered 'reasonable' by both the employee and the employer.

Such adjustments could include:

- allowing the employee to work from home
- providing longer break periods
- providing ramps and wheelchair access
- transferring the employee to a role with fewer physical demands.

Different countries have different laws to protect people with MS from discrimination on the basis of their disability (see Useful resources, page 131). Some laws also cover people who are the primary carers for people with MS.

Key points – lifestyle considerations and the multidisciplinary team

- Counseling is helpful for all people with multiple sclerosis (MS): it will involve explaining the nature of the disease, the risks and benefits of therapy, and the impact MS will have on all aspects of life, including career, family, travel and insurance.
- Common concerns raised by patients include life expectancy, heritability of the disease and effect of pregnancy.
- A multidisciplinary team is important for the coordination of patient care, and comprises neurologists, family practitioners, specialist nurses, physiotherapists, speech and language therapists, occupational therapists, dietitians, social workers, psychologists and continence nurses.
- Specialist MS nurses are a reliable source of information about all aspects of the condition. They have an important role in helping patients recognize the signs and symptoms of relapse, providing practical advice on living with MS and providing a link with other services.
- Concerns about employment can become a great source of stress. Employers have an obligation to aid people with MS as much as possible to remain in employment.

Driving

If a job involves driving, employers must be informed of the MS diagnosis. In the UK, people with a driving licence who have been diagnosed with MS must tell the Driver and Vehicle Licensing Agency (DVLA). In Australia, the relevant authority in each state must be informed. The driving authority may then contact the patient's doctor, and will decide on a case-by-case basis. In the USA, people with MS may need to be assessed by a member of the Association for Driver Rehabilitation Specialists. They will either recommend no driving, adaptations to be made to the car to assist driving, or unrestricted driving, depending on the results of a full assessment including input from the medical team.

Key references

Australia: Disability Discrimination Act
http://www.hreoc.gov.au/disability_rights/dda_guide/areas/areas.html

NICE. *Clinical Guidance 8: Management of multiple sclerosis in primary and secondary care.* London: National Institute for Health and Care Excellence, November 2003. http://guidance.nice.org.uk/CG8, last accessed 12 March 2014.

UK: Equality Act and the Disability Discrimination Act http://webarchive.nationalarchives.gov.uk/+/www.direct.gov.uk/en/DisabledPeople/RightsAndObligations/DisabilityRights/DG_4001068

US Americans with Disabilities Act (1990)
http://www.ada.gov/

Mortality

Multiple sclerosis (MS) can almost span a lifetime: average time from disease onset to death is 48 years. Natural history studies suggest that people with MS have a reduced life expectancy of approximately 6–7 years, and the mortality rate is three times higher than that of the general population. Women tend to survive longer than men, unless they have the primary progressive subtype, in which case they do less well than men. Disease onset at a younger age is also associated with longer survival.

Use of immunomodulatory drugs (Chapter 5) may reduce time to secondary progression, and there is soft evidence of a positive effect on all-cause mortality from the long term (21-year) follow up of patients randomized to interferon beta-1b in the pivotal Phase III trial of that therapy.

Death is usually caused by a complication rather than as a direct result of a MS exacerbation (Table 9.1).

Aspects of disease progression

The course of MS is highly variable and often unpredictable in the early relapsing phase of the disease. However, secondary progression ensues in up to 75% of patients with relapsing remitting disease and is marked by inexorable decline that is unaffected by current treatments.

TABLE 9.1

Causes of death in multiple sclerosis

- Cardiovascular disease
- Cancer
- Infection (urinary sepsis, aspiration pneumonia, skin sores)
- Accident/suicide

In a proportion of these patients, severe symptomatology affecting all aspects of neurological functioning may develop. A cohesive multidisciplinary team (see Chapter 8) is important to effectively manage this phase of the disease. Neuropsychiatric complications, including depression and cognitive impairment, can limit or impede interactions with healthcare services.

Common features of advanced MS include:
- dysphagia
- recurrent infections (urinary tract or aspiration pneumonia)
- Expanded Disability Status Score (EDSS) above 8.0 (bedbound) – see Table 3.9, page 52
- cognitive decline
- weight loss.

Palliative care

Early intervention from the palliative care team can be highly beneficial to the patient's quality of life. As far as possible, control over the effects of the disease process should remain with the patient.

The World Health Organization states that palliative care is an approach that improves the quality of life of patients and families facing the problems associated with life-threatening illness, through the prevention and relief of suffering by means of early identification and impeccable assessment and treatment of pain and other problems – physical, psychosocial and spiritual. Spiritual beliefs are not necessarily related to religion, although for many people their faiths, beliefs and practices will be important. Spirituality has many facets, for example questions concerning identity, the meaning of life, suffering and death, and reconciliation and forgiveness. While it is important that any needs in this respect are identified and provided for, it is not always appropriate within the healthcare setting. There may be a role for local chaplaincy services (for any religion) or support from psychological services.

Palliative care is commonly perceived as a type of care only available at the end stages of a disease, usually cancer. Today, the focus is on integration of palliative care with ongoing treatment.

TABLE 9.2

Aspects of MS that may benefit from palliative care

- Pain control
- Anxiety/depression
- Oral care
- Skin integrity and risk of pressure sores

- Feeding
- Continence
- Spasms
- Bowel problems

Discussion of the results of disease progression and possible outcomes can be valuable. It can facilitate planning for the future, and consideration of complex decisions, when there is enough time for clear evaluation.

Aspects of MS that may benefit from the input of the palliative care team are shown in Table 9.2. Palliative care in people with MS is not typical of palliative care in patients with other conditions in that it can be introduced in patients who are still receiving active treatment. It can be perceived as care of the dying patient, but this is a limiting perspective that prevents the benefits of palliative care reaching a wider group of patients.

End-stage MS can be managed at home with specialist nursing care, or in a hospital or hospice.

Pressure sores. People with MS who are no longer mobile are at risk of developing pressure sores. It is important to monitor, and regularly inspect, vulnerable areas such as the sacrum, heels and medial malleoli. In patients with contractures, inspection of the areas under constant pressure is vital.

Multidisciplinary management should involve the dietitian to ensure there is adequate nutrition to maintain healthy skin, as well as the tissue viability specialist team who will advise on mattresses, cushions and appropriate dressings to help to minimize the risk of pressure sore development.

Feeding. Aspiration pneumonia can become a problem when swallowing becomes impaired. Help from speech and language therapists and dietitians can minimize this risk. When dysphagia, apathy from depression or cognitive impairment develops, people with MS may not be able to maintain their nutritional intake. It is then that percutaneous enteral gastrostomy should be considered (PEG feeding). However, the decision to proceed with PEG feeding is complex and reflects the individual's experience and quality of life. This decision is often included in an advance directive.

Continence. Bladder problems arising from MS are often exacerbated by limited mobility and coordination, which makes self-catheterization difficult. In later stages, insertion of suprapubic catheters may be the treatment of choice. Before inserting a catheter, the patient should be formally assessed by a continence specialist. The plan to insert a suprapubic catheter may be driven by recurrent urinary tract infection and symptoms despite maximal drug therapy. In the community, regular assessment by skilled nurses is essential, to maintain function and to minimize infection.

Advance directives

These are legal documents that inform the professionals caring for a person with MS what their wishes would be in a variety of situations. As individuals may reach a point where they are no longer deemed to have the capacity to make decisions about their own care, these decisions clearly need to be made in advance. The legal power of these documents varies from one jurisdiction to another, but advance directives are a vital part of the decision-making process (Table 9.3)

Power of attorney

Lasting (UK), enduring (Australia) or durable (USA) power of attorney is an alternative to an advance directive, whereby a person with MS can appoint a person (spouse, parent, sibling) to make decisions regarding their care once they are no longer able to. This can include decisions regarding their finances and well-being, as well as specific healthcare decisions.

TABLE 9.3

Examples of decisions that can be included in an advance directive

- Parenteral feeding
- Catheterization
- Treatment of infection
- Resuscitation after cardiac arrest

Key points – advanced multiple sclerosis

- Natural history studies suggest that life expectancy of people with multiple sclerosis (MS) is reduced by 6–7 years compared with unaffected individuals.
- The average time from disease onset to mortality is 48 years.
- Early introduction of disease-modifying therapy may positively effect long-term mortality.
- Palliative care offers patients improved quality of life in the later stages of the disease.
- Advance planning can help people with MS achieve the control they need in late disease.

Key references

Culliford L. Spiritual care and psychiatric treatment: an introduction. *Adv Psychiatr Treat* 2002;8:249–58. http://apt.rcpsych.org/content/8/4/249.full, last accessed 12 March 2014.

Degenhardt A, Ramagopalan SV, Scalfari A, Ebers GC. Clinical prognostic factors in multiple sclerosis: a natural history review. *Nat Rev Neurol* 2009;5:672–82.

Ebers GC. Natural history of multiple sclerosis. *J Neurol Neurosurg Psychiatry* 2001;71(suppl 2):ii16–19.

Edmonds P, Hart S, Gao W et al. Palliative care for people severely affected by multiple sclerosis: evaluation of a novel palliative care service. *Mult Scler* 2010;16:627–36.

Gruenewald DA, Higginson IJ, Vivat B et al. Quality of life measures for the palliative care of people severely affected by multiple sclerosis: a systematic review. *Mult Scler* 2004;10:690–704.

Multiple Sclerosis Society. MS and palliative care: a guide for health and social care professionals. Multiple Sclerosis Society, 2006. www.mssociety.org.uk/sites/default/files/Documents/Professionals/MS%20and%20Palliative%20Care%20-%20guide%20for%20professionals.pdf, last accessed 12 March 2014.

National Council for Palliative Care, Neurological Alliance, National End of Life Care Programme. End of life care in long term neurological conditions – a framework for implementation. Crown Copyright, 2011. www.mssociety.org.uk/ms-resources/end-life-care-long-term-neurological-conditions-%E2%80%93-framework-implementation, last accessed 12 March 2014.

Useful resources

UK

Action MS – Northern Ireland
Tel: +44 (0)28 9079 0707
info@actionms.co.uk
www.xiportal.com/actionms

Association of British Neurologists
Tel: +44 (0)20 7405 4060
info@theabn.org
www.theabn.org

British Association/College of Occupational Therapists
Tel: +44 (0)20 7357 6480
Reception@cot.co.uk
www.cot.co.uk

Capability Scotland
Tel: +44 (0)131 337 9876
www.capability-scotland.org.uk

Carers UK
Adviceline: 0808 808 7777
Tel: +44 (0)20 7378 4999
adviceline@carersuk.org
www.carersuk.org

Chartered Society of Physiotherapy
Tel: +44 (0)20 7306 6666
www.csp.org.uk

Connect
The Communication Disability Network
Tel: +44 (0)20 7367 0840
info@ukconnect.org
www.ukconnect.org

Dial Network (Scope)
Scope response: 0808 800 3333
response@scope.org.uk
www.scope.org.uk/dial

Disability Rights UK
Tel: +44 (0)20 7250 3222
enquiries@disabilityrightsuk.org
http://disabilityrightsuk.org

Disability Wales
Tel: +44 (0)29 2088 7325
info@disabilitywales.org
www.disabilitywales.org

Disabled Living Foundation
Helpline: 0300 999 0004
helpline@dlf.org.uk
info@dlf.org.uk
www.dlf.org.uk

Forum of Mobility Centres
Toll-free: 0800 559 3636
mobility@rcht.cornwall.nhs.uk
www.mobility-centres.org.uk

MS-UK
Toll-free: 0800 783 0518
Tel: +44 (0)1206 226500
www.ms-uk.org

Multiple Sclerosis National
Therapy Centres
Tel: 0845 367 0977
info@msntc.org.uk
www.msntc.org.uk

Multiple Sclerosis Society
Tel: +44 (0)20 8438 0700
helpline@mssociety.org.uk
infoteam@mssociety.org.uk
www.mssociety.org.uk

Multiple Sclerosis Trust
Toll-free: 0800 032 3839
info@mstrust.org.uk
www.mstrust.org.uk

The Neurological Alliance
Tel: +44 (0)20 7584 6457
admin@neural.org.uk
www.neural.org.uk

Primary Care Neurology Society
Tel: +44 (0)20 3479 5111
info@p-cns.org.uk
www.p-cns.org.uk

Speakability
Helpline: 080 8808 9572
speakability@speakability.org.uk
www.speakability.org.uk

USA
American Academy of Neurology
Toll-free: 800 879 1960
Tel: +1 612 928 6000
www.aan.com

American Neurological
Association
Tel: +1 856 638 0423
www.aneuroa.org

The Consortium of Multiple
Sclerosis Centers
Tel: +1 201 487 1050
www.mscare.org

Multiple Sclerosis Association of
America
Toll-free: 800 532 7667
MSquestions@mymsaa.org
www.mymsaa.org

Multiple Sclerosis Foundation
Toll-free: 888 673 6287
support@msfocus.org
www.msfocus.org

National Institute of Neurological
Disorders and Stroke
Toll-free: 800 352 9424
www.ninds.nih.gov

National Multiple Sclerosis
Society
Toll-free: 1 800 344 4867
www.nationalmssociety.org

International

European Committee for Treatment and Research in Multiple Sclerosis (ECTRIMS)
Tel: +41 (0)61 686 77 79
secretariat@ectrims.eu
www.ectrims.eu

MS Australia
Tel: +61 (0)2 8484 1315
info@msaustralia.org.au
www.msaustralia.org.au

MS Research Australia
Tel: 1300 356 467
www.msra.org.au

Multiple Sclerosis International Federation
Tel: +44 (0)20 7620 1911
www.msif.org

Multiple Sclerosis Society of Canada
Tel: +1 416 922 6065
info@mssociety.ca
http://mssociety.ca

Multiple Sclerosis South Africa
Tel: +27 (0)21 948 4160
http://multiplesclerosis.co.za

Pan-Asian Committee for Treatment and Research in Multiple Sclerosis (PACTRIMS)
secretariat@pactrims.org
www.pactrims.org

Further reading at fastfacts.com
Fast Facts: Bladder Disorders
Fast Facts: Chronic and Cancer Pain
Fast Facts: Dementia
Fast Facts: Depression
Fast Facts: Epilepsy
Fast Facts: Parkinson's Disease

FastTest

You've read the book ... now test yourself with key questions from the authors
***FREE* at fastfacts.com**

- Go to: www.fastfacts.com/fast-facts/Multiple-Sclerosis-3rd-edn
- Click on the ***FastTest*** to open the interactive PDF

Index

activities of daily living 70, 120–1
acute disseminated encephalomyelitis (ADEM) 17, 46–7, 110–11, 112
adolescents 110, 113
advance directives 128
advanced disease 125–9
alemtuzumab 84, 94, 98–9
alternative therapies 119
amantadine 63
amitryptiline 67, 68
analgesia 67, 68
anesthetics 118
antibody tests *see* immunoglobulin tests
anticonvulsants 67, 68, 72
antidepressants 67, 68
anti-LINGO antibody 22, 103
aquaporin 4 (AQP-4) 45, 112
autoimmune diseases 31, 47
iatrogenic 99
azathioprine 45, 93, 108

baclofen, oral 60, 61, 67
baclofen pumps 62, 63
benign MS 29–30
benzodiazepines 60, 61
bladder problems 34–5, 64–7, 108, 121, 128
blood tests
diagnosis 40, 45, 112–13
monitoring 81, 115
bone loss 58, 121
bone marrow transplantation 95, 101–2
botulinum toxin 60–2, 66–7
bowel problems 35, 67
breastfeeding 108
burning pain 34, 68

cannabinoids 60, 68
carbamazepine 67, 68, 72

cardiac side effects 86, 115
catheterization 64, 65, 67, 128
cerebrospinal fluid (CSF) 41, 112
children 46–7, 110–15
clinical cases 43, 63, 77, 78, 83, 89
clinically definite MS 25
clinically isolated syndrome (CIS) 25, 76, 77–8
cognitive behavioral therapy 63
cognitive impairment 36, 113, 126
constipation 35, 67, 121
contraception 107, 113
corpus callosum 15, 50, 112
cortical lesions 15, 16, 22, 36, 40, 72
corticosteroids 47, 49, 58–9, 68, 107, 114
counseling 117, 118–19
cyclophosphamide 93, 95

daclizumab 100
dantrolene 60, 61
demyelination 17, 18–19, 22
dental procedures 118
depression 36, 63, 72, 115, 126
desmopressin 65
detrusor hyperactivity 35, 64–6
diagnosis 25, 37–43, 56, 112–13
differentials 40, 43–50, 110–11
diarrhea 67
diazepam 60, 61
diet 67, 118, 121, 127, 128
vitamin D 9–10, 103
dimethyl fumarate 91–2, 107

disability 33–4, 50–5, 69, 113, 122–3
discrimination 122–3
disease-modifying therapies 45, 75–101, 107–8, 114, 115
driving 72, 124
duloxetine 68
dysarthria 33, 120
dysphagia 33, 120, 128

early relapsing MS 18, 21, 22, 75
elderly patients 115–16
electrophysiology 41–2, 113
employment 50–1, 122–3
encephalopathy 46–7, 110
enteral feeding 120, 121, 128
environmental risk factors 9–10
ephaptic transmission 34, 67
epidemiology 7–10, 11, 12, 49, 110, 125
epilepsy 70, 72, 113
Epstein Barr virus 10
ethnicity 7, 13, 49
etiology 7
Expanded Disability Status Scale (EDSS) 51–3, 113

falls 69, 115
family history 31
fampridine 19, 70
fatigue 62–4, 113
females 9, 10, 106–9, 110
fingolimod 45, 84–7, 107, 115
flu-like side effects 81
flushing 92, 114
functional electrical stimulation 71

gabapentin 60, 61, 67, 68
gadolinium-enhancing lesions 39, 44, 49

gait 33, 69–71
gender 9, 10, 110
genetics 9, 10–13
geographical distribution
8–9
glatiramer acetate 76–80,
94, 107, 114
gray matter lesions 15, 16,
22, 36, 40, 72

heat 31, 59
history 30–1
home adaptations 70,
120–1
human leukocyte antigen
(HLA) 9, 11–12
hypertension 108–9

immunization 32, 118
immunoglobulin,
intravenous 47, 114
immunoglobulin tests
CSF 41, 112
serum 40, 45, 112
immunosuppressants 45,
92–3, 95, 108, 115
immunotherapy
disease-modifying 45,
75–101, 107–8, 114, 115
remyelination 22, 103
incidence 8
incontinence
fecal 67
urinary 34–5, 64–7, 108,
121, 128
infections 10, 31–2, 59,
84, 86, 99, 108, 112–13
inflammation 15–19, 22,
37, 39, 40, 68
injections 78–9, 99
interferon beta 45, 76–82,
94, 107, 114, 115
internuclear
ophthalmoplegia 32–3

JC virus 40, 84

lamotrigine 67, 68, 72
laquinimod 100–1
late-onset MS 115
legal issues 122–3, 124, 128

L'hermitte's sign 30, 67–8
lifestyle 70, 117, 120–3
liver function 81, 90, 114

McDonald diagnostic
criteria 42–3, 44–5
macrophages 18
males 9, 10, 110
management 73, 96, 104
of children 113–15
dietary 67, 103, 121, 128
disease-modifying
therapies 75–101, 107–8,
114, 115
of the elderly 115
monitoring therapy 40,
81, 84, 115
multidisciplinary 69,
113, 115, 117–21, 123,
127
of NMO 45, 100
palliative care 126–8
in pregnancy 107–8
of relapses 58–9, 107,
114
remyelination 22, 103
stem cells 95, 101–2
by subtype 25–6, 94–5
of symptoms 59–72
timing 75–6, 78, 81–2,
94–5
men 9, 10
mesenchymal stem cells 102
methotrexate 108
methylprednisolone 59,
107, 114
microglia 18, 19
migraine 68
migration studies 10
mitoxantrone 93
mobility 33, 34, 69–71,
108, 120
modafinil 63–4
monitoring
progression 51–5
therapy 40, 81, 84, 115
mood disorders 36, 63,
72, 115, 126
mortality 125
motor symptoms 33, 34,
115

movement disorders 33–4,
60–2, 67, 72
MRI (magnetic resonance
imaging)
MS 37–40, 53–5, 78, 84,
112
NMO 48–9
sarcoidosis 49–50
multidisciplinary teams
69, 113, 115, 117–21,
123, 127
muscular problems 33–4,
60–2, 67, 72
mycophenolate 45

nabilone 60
nabiximols 60
natalizumab 40, 82–4, 94,
107, 114
natural history 28, 50,
125–6
neurodegeneration 22, 54
neurologists 117
neuromyelitis optica
(NMO) 43–6, 67, 100,
111
neuropathic pain 34, 68–9
nortryptiline 67, 68
nurses 119–20

occupational therapists
120–1
ocrelizumab 99–100
ofatumumab 99–100
oligoclonal bands 41, 112
oligodendrocytes 17, 19,
21, 103
optic neuritis 15, 32, 43–6,
59, 68, 111
orthotic devices 70, 71
oxybutynin 64–5
oxygen therapy 119

pain 34, 67–9
palliative care 126–8
paresis 34
paresthesia 34, 68
pathology 15–23
pediatrics 46–7, 110–15
physiotherapy 69–70, 120
posture 34

power of attorney 128
prednisolone/prednisone 59
pregabalin 67, 68
pregnancy 90, 106–9, 113, 118
presentation 25, 30–6, 56, 110, 115
pressure sores 127
prevalence 7, 8–9, 11
primary care providers 117–19
primary progressive MS 28, 115
prognosis 50–5, 78, 111, 113
progression 27–8, 51–4, 106, 125
progressive multifocal leukoencephalopathy (PML) 40, 84, 92
progressive relapsing MS 29

race 7, 13, 49
refractory disease 92–3, 94–5, 101–2
relapses 18–19, 31–2, 106
management 58–9, 107, 114
relapsing remitting MS 26, 54, 110
management 75–103
remission 26
remyelination 19–22, 103
rhizotomy 62
risk factors
initial 9–13
for progression 27, 78, 111
rituximab 45, 99–100

sarcoidosis 40, 47–9
season of birth effect 9
secondary progressive MS 16, 27, 54, 93, 98, 113, 125–6
seizures 70, 72, 113
sensory symptoms 34, 68
sex (gender) 9, 10, 110
sexual dysfunction 36, 106
signs and symptoms 30–6, 47, 56, 110, 113, 115
management 59–72
smoking 10
social history 31
social support 113, 115, 120
social workers 121
solifenacin 64–5
spasticity 33–4, 60–2, 67
specialist nurses 119–20
speech problems 33, 120
spinal cord disease 15, 30, 31, 34, 35, 39–40, 48, 108–9
spiritual beliefs 126
stem cell therapies 95, 101–2
stereotactic surgery 69
steroids 47, 49, 58–9, 68, 107, 114
subtypes 25–30
suicide 115
swallowing problems 33, 120, 128
symptoms 31–6, 47, 110, 113, 115
management 59–72
systemic autoimmunity 47

T cells 15, 18, 76, 88, 98, 106
teratogens 90, 108
teriflunomide 88–91, 108
thromboprophylaxis 108
tizanidine 60, 61
tolterodine 64–5
treatment see management
tricyclic antidepressants 67, 68
trigeminal neuralgia 34, 67
twins 11

Uhthoff's phenomenon 31, 59
ultrasound 34–5
ultraviolet radiation 9
urinary problems 34–5, 64–7, 108, 121, 128

vaccination 32, 118
visual defects 32–3
visual evoked potentials 42
vitamin D 9–10, 103, 106

walking 33, 69–71
weakness 34
white matter
degeneration 22, 54
periplaque 19
plaques 15–19, 37
remyelination 19–22, 103
women 9, 10, 106–9

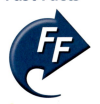

Fast Facts:
Multiple Sclerosis

Third edition

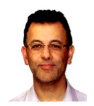

Omar Malik PhD FRCP
Consultant Neurologist and Honorary Clinical Senior Lecturer
Imperial College Healthcare NHS Trust
Department of Neurology
Charing Cross Hospital
London, UK

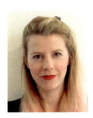

Ann Donnelly MRCP
Specialty Registrar
Department of Neurology
Kings College Hospital
London, UK

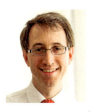

Michael Barnett MB BS FRACP PhD
Associate Professor in Neurology and
Consultant Neurologist
Royal Prince Alfred Hospital and
The Brain & Mind Research Institute
Sydney, Australia

Declaration of Independence
This book is as balanced and as practical as we can make it.
Ideas for improvement are always welcome: feedback@fastfacts.com

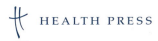

HEALTH PRESS

Fast Facts: Multiple Sclerosis
First published 2000; second edition 2006
Third edition April 2014

Text © 2014 Omar Malik, Ann Donnelly, Michael Barnett
© 2014 in this edition Health Press Limited

Health Press Limited, Elizabeth House, Queen Street, Abingdon,
Oxford OX14 3LN, UK
Tel: +44 (0)1235 523233
Fax: +44 (0)1235 523238
Book orders can be placed by telephone or via the website.
For regional distributors or to order via the website, please go to: fastfacts.com
For telephone orders, please call +44 (0)1752 202301 (UK, Europe and Asia–
Pacific), 1 800 247 6553 (USA, toll free) or +1 419 281 1802 (Americas).

Fast Facts is a trademark of Health Press Limited.

A CIP record for this title is available from the British Library.

ISBN 978-1-908541-33-8

Malik O (Omar)
Fast Facts: Multiple Sclerosis/
Omar Malik, Ann Donnelly, Michael Barnett

Cover image: Colored sagittal fluid-attenuated inversion recovery MRI scan
showing globular and pericallosal lesions in a patient with MS.

Medical illustrations by Annamaria Dutto, Withernsea, UK.
Typesetting and page layout by Zed, Oxford, UK.
Printed in China.